# THE STRESS AFFECT

## HOW TO RESCUE YOUR LIFE AND MASTER THE ART OF LIVING

## Dr. Nigel Brayer

THE STRESS AFFECT
HOW TO RESCUE YOUR LIFE AND MASTER THE ART OF LIVING
ISBN: 978-0-9903960-7-9
By Dr. Nigel Brayer

1st Printing, August 2014
Printed in the United States of America

# Dedication

---

To all of my patients, friends, my loving and supportive wife Brandi and my children Nicholas, Celeste, Seth and Jude. I Thank You for giving me the experiences in life that have allowed me to create this book. Through living, clinical practice, being a husband, father and participant in the cyclical flow of life I give you my observations, of what I have observed works and what does not, why disease is created and how it is stopped or reversed. I share with you as a clinician, but more importantly as one who is also seeking a greater level of health, longevity, vitality and peace, and one who himself is learning the best possible way to live, to be healthy and to live peacefully.

To all of you I will never meet, I hope my experiences and words can help broaden your understanding, give you hope and initiate some positive change in your life. This is my goal and purpose, to make your life a little better off than before we met, either personally or through these words.

Some of you may read these words and get angry and frustrated; know that how you respond to this information is yours and yours alone. Some may say I am against modern medicine, pharmaceuticals and surgery.  That would be untrue also. I am an absolute advocate for the use of these tools as a last resort to managing what can no longer be improved by supporting the body, and letting its natural powers do the work.

One of my greatest desires with the production of this book will be to help the world, which includes me, to "WAKE UP" to itself. Wake up to the diseases we are creating, wake up before our only options are to "MANAGE the symptoms of disease" with chemicals that will always create more disease. Finally my desire is to restore faith in "You," yes, you as a person, you as a city of billions of cells, cells that form communities, have transportation and communication lines, special strengths and weakness and are run by a mysterious power that made YOU...from two cells. A you that responds and adapts without your awareness of it. My wish, to restore faith in the power that "BREATHED" life into those two cells that grew into the magnificent world contained by your outer flesh, a world that you have the power to destroy or to heal, through your thoughts, your words and your actions.

If I could restore just a little faith back into the MIRACLE of our bodies and remind us that our bodies ARE miracles, we could start living with an air of gratitude and reverence. This would change our minds, our choices and our lives. This simple shift changes all the variables. Remember we are all the same, we all desire health, we all desire joy, we all desire peace. However, in my observation, we are all looking in the wrong direction. Imagine what would happen individually and globally if we started simply beholding the grandeur of our most prized possession, our body. Imagine if we stopped waiting for someone, or something, to save us and have faith that with a little understanding and a few regular habit changes we can change ourselves. Is technology useful?  Of course! Are doctors useful? Of course!  Are medications useful? Of course! However, we need to remember that our body knows what to do to heal a wound on our finger if we just give the body what it needs, leave it alone and let the magic happen.

"If you don't go within, you a simply go without!" - Victor Frankl

We have all spent most of our lives looking for answers outside of ourselves; perhaps it's time to go within? This book is for those.

# Contents

# Foreword

---

The bucket list has become a modern ICON of our final days, the list of what we want to do when we know our time has come. A list of all of the things in our life that we have put on hold and just couldn't get around to due to the distractions, responsibilities and obligations of life. The movie that many of us have laughed with gives us an impression of how things get away from us. For those who have not watched the movie, the basic premise is this: life builds up, gets in the way of the direction we want our life to take. The directions we actually end up taking are rarely the same. In the movie the characters decide to right that and the adventure begins.

In the coming pages we are going to redefine for you the bucket effect of life. Instead of getting crazy at our final hour to make up for lost time we will discuss how life accumulates, how it affects our life and creates our health or disease experience. Most importantly, we will learn how we can change the outcomes in our life. This book's purpose is to give every person who reads it a simple understanding of cause and effect, energy/effort and resistance, stress and balance. The primary purpose is to **Encourage** you to move forward, **Enrich** your life with new perspectives and finally find **Inspiration** to move in a direction of health, happiness and peace.

Imagine for a moment... each of us is allotted a certain amount of energy. Imagine this as a bucket, some bigger, some smaller. Each person may have more or less than others, based upon genetics, disposition, physical attributes, etc. However, that bucket represents the energy that is available to us, for living life, breathing, digesting, exercising, healing, work, play, kids and whatever else constitutes your life. On that bucket is a line, for our purposes let's call it a threshold, an arbitrary line that is different for everyone. It can be anywhere on that bucket. For some it's higher or lower than for others, based upon the element above (genetics, disposition etc). We can call this line, imbalance for some, symptoms for another, disease for others or any other effect of the body's inability to maintain balance. For our purposes let's call it an awareness that something isn't in right inside of you, or even a symptom of some sort.

Now, imagine all of the conscious (you are aware of them) and unconscious (you are not aware of them) challenges in our life that suck up some of that energy in your bucket. When this occurs the energy level in your bucket drops closer to the line as mentioned above, the symptom or disease line. Now imagine next we do things in our life to add energy back into the bucket, for instance learning new ways of living, new habits, new behaviors. These new ways then add energy or volume back into your bucket. If you stay above this individual threshold as we spoke of earlier, you will experience more of the effect of balance. Meaning your body would be generally functional, you would have fewer symptoms and your likelihood of disease is lower than it would be then if you were at or below the threshold line. Remember that each person's LINE is different than others. Therefore what may cause symptoms or disease in one may not cause the same level of symptoms or disease in another.

As we proceed, I am going to challenge you to look at every part of your life as either adding to your bucket of life energy and balance or taking it away. You will question much of this book because you have been conditioned to think that life is complicated, the body is confusing and diseases need to be attacked. I am going to challenge you to take a broader approach to the common conundrums of our species and not ask yourself, "Why did this happen to me?" but rather, "How did I create the environment to which my body is now in, and more importantly, how can I un-create what I don't want and create what I do?" With this knowledge and a few simple tools we will lay out a path to change. This change will come first by understanding, second by action and finally will produce results. Different than the ones you are now living.

For some of you this will sound too good to be true or you will write this new information off as a fad or gimmick. I pray this is not your approach, for no action is action to continue on the path you are on. If your life and health are exactly how you want it then perfect, carry on. If not, then you are missing a very big opportunity to achieve what you desire. For others, you may believe these simple steps to regain balance in your life are "too simple," for again we have been conditioned to believe that you must be a genius to figure out the inner workings of the body. Of course this isn't true. However, if it were true about all of life that would mean we would have to be an electronics genius to be able to run a computer or use a cell phone. Our body is like a computer or phone; we do not need to be a master of its intricacies like neuroanatomy, psychology, biochemistry or physiology to create health and well being. We need only understand a few basic operations to navigate in the right direction.

Throughout this book we will ask you to remember and in time convince yourself that life is simple, and in time you will begin to believe that life is simple for the most part, with a few complications here and there to keep us interested.

Finally, there will be a few of you who will disregard all parts of this book because your conditioning of the complexities of life is so ingrained that a perspective other than the one you know is not possible. You may even become angry and send notes of your disgust at the prospect that your entire belief system about health and disease is being challenged. That is OK. The intent of this book is not to throw any of you into a place where all of your founding beliefs are thrown on the chopping block. Rather, it is to give those who are open a perspective that they may not have considered or to affirm what perhaps deep down you always knew but didn't allow yourself to believe and live.

Whatever your reasoning for reading this book, my sincerest wish is that you find Encouragement to continue to move forward in whatever direction you chose, Enrichment through a deeper understanding of the universal laws of nature and Inspiration to learn, to hope, to build faith and to create peace, first within yourself and then into the world.

# 1

## We Are All the Same

Have you ever considered our sameness? Our world has become incredibly proficient at identifying our differences, yet have you really ever considered how alike we all are? The Middle East, Asia, Africa, North America, South America, East, West, Black, White, Spanish, Caucasian, Baptists, Atheists, Muslims, Christians, Vegans, Carnivores, Fat, Thin, Strong, Weak, Gay, Straight, Republican, Democrat. Every one of these examples creates an instantaneous response of our differences, which yes do exist, yet our Sameness is so much greater.

We have all heard that what we look for we find. Sadly, I have observed that most of our world has conditioned us to find our differences, which in turn increases our separation from each other. This separation of course creates resistance, conflict and barriers. Does this mean that we must always be in agreement? Of course this is not possible; however, an understanding of our ingrained pattern of creating barriers will be key as we progress in the understanding of our greatest barrier – "ourselves" – and more importantly, the internal responses we create within ourselves, which result in either an experience of Health or the experience of disease. As we progress many of us will wonder, "What does our responses to our differences have to do with health?" The answer will always be the same. Everything! How we respond to anything creates an effect on everything within our body, and most importantly our cells. Our responses can be differentiated into two groups. 1. They create ease, cooperation and health or 2. They create friction, resistance or disease. As confusing as it all sounds virtually every aspect, every action, every food and every thought can be categorized as supporting or resisting. If our focus is on differences we have a tendency to create within ourselves resistance or protection. When our focus is on similarities our tendency tends toward progression and cooperation. Of course there will be many exceptions, however, for our purposes it is extremely important to understand our physical responses. These responses whether we are aware of them or not affect our biology, immediately and temporarily, and eventually permanently. As our biology, or our cell actions change in time, our experiences change, from the experience of health to the experience of disease.

EXERCISE: Think of an experience that makes you extremely happy, think about the details, the components that make you glad, the events or the people involved. Bask in that moment for awhile. How do you feel? Do you feel light, at ease, at peace? These responses create relaxation, ease, healing and growth. Does this make your day easier or more difficult? Imagine if you could be in this state of no resistance constantly. How would your life be different?

Now imagine a circumstance in your past or present that makes you extremely angry. Without letting it ruin your whole day, look into that experience a little bit; observe you physical reaction. Are your muscles tensing? Perhaps your shoulders are getting closer to your ears. Feel the tension rising. This is resistance. Does this make your day easier or more difficult? Imagine if you could be in this state of resistance constantly, how would your life be different?

The higher the resistance, the more energy required to overcome the resistance.

We call this the emergency brake effect. When your emergency brake is on it takes a lot more energy from the car's motor to keep it moving. Now remember the bucket effect. How much energy in your life is being used countering resistance? And how much is left for living, healing and building?

How are you creating resistance in your life? We are all creating a great deal. However, the relative amounts will create the flow, or direction in your life, and the experiences you experience. This includes the symptoms or conditions in your life.

## CHANGE CREATES GROWTH/ACCEPTANCE CREATES PEACE

It is no doubt, and most of us can relate that life creates an abundance of challenges that we must confront daily. There are scheduling conflicts, co-worker challenges, work deadlines, do or die business deals, relationship resistance, and of course then there's parenting.

This is definitely not an all-inclusive list. I am certain you have many challenges that were not listed above. However, one thing is certain. These challenges will never go away, they will continue indefinitely, so where does that leave us? For many, it's being frustrated, overwhelmed, sleepless, medicated and sadly diseased. If that was the whole story as most of our world believes we are left dressing wounds, treating symptoms, performing reactionary surgeries and holding on day by day, asking ourselves if this is what life is about. Thank goodness that's only half of the story!

What if the outcome could be different? I have observed now in nearly 17 years in practice that most of us have exhausted the old way of living. We are all too tired to keep pushing down the same path, doing the same thing and expecting different results. We have had it with hitting our heads against the same wall. I have observed that many of us are tired of the pain that comes from staying in the same rut and are ready to move past the fear and temporary pain resulting from change. We are ready to jump into the unknown with the prospect of getting what we have always desired, but did not believe it possible. What's most interesting is this is a self discovery. No one can make this discovery for you, and no one but you can decide what direction you wish to go.

I see an overwhelming number of people who are now willing to embrace change rather than resist it. The result is always growth and some form of a new direction. No one said it is easy! Our patterns of behavior are "OURS." We have created them, usually unconsciously, meaning we didn't necessarily decide to choose our behaviors; rather they were created one at a time over a lifetime. They were created as a means of navigating our world, getting our needs met and making sense of things based upon our understanding at the time. What's different now? You! You have the opportunity now to decide which life habits or perspectives serve your goals and which do not, and what experiences we chose to live in the future, more of the same, or something different.

Each of our habits and perspectives are based upon hundreds, maybe thousands, of factors which Freud spent his lifetime analyzing and evaluating. None of that is important for the purposes of change that we will be embarking on in the coming pages. However, the important part most of us need to understand is that, we have patterns of behavior. Those patterns are our DEFAULT settings for how we think, how we act and of course what we experience. This applies whether it be financially, how we experience relationships with others, ourselves and of course what we experience at the level of physical health. All of these experiences can be considered an outcome or an effect of our self-created patterns or interactions with the world.

Outcomes you say? You got it! What we are experiencing today good, bad or in between are the outcomes of our interactions, of all the facets of life. This book is about changing the outcomes, as it applies to our bodies, and our experiences of health or disease. It could however just as easily be a book on relationships, business or raising well adjusted responsible and independent children. Results are outcomes. Results are never the problem, although they can certainly cause us all a lot of suffering. To understand this concept fully you need only ask yourself the question. If I remove all of the outcomes or results I do not want in my life will I solve the problem? Reflect on this for a moment. If I remove all of the alcohol in the world will I stop alcoholism? Did prohibition work? If I remove all of the drugs in the world will we stop addiction? How about this, if I find a cure for cancer, will I stop cancer's occurrence in the body. I believe if you look honestly at the question you will have to agree that the solutions to most of our health problems, and in many cases life problems, cannot be resolved by trying to change the symptom. Has modern Western medicine stopped the effects of diseases? We could say yes. The symptoms have been impacted differently than say 100 years ago. Medicines have helped alleviate many symptoms better. Our technologies have improved identification and earlier detection of disease process and have certainly kept people alive longer. These are great advances but have any of them really changed the causes? For instance, what causes the environment within our body to allow cancer to occur? Why does inflammation build and cause destruction of the joints, blood vessels and nerves? Consider all of it and what created the outcome.

Symptoms are results, like two plus two equals four. What if you falsely made the result different? We know that two plus two equals four, however when your child makes a mistake in the equation and says two plus two equals seven, we do not miraculously erase the answer for them to make them feel better, in this case the wrong answer of seven. As a parent we go back to the factors in the equation, we know the answer lies within these factors, not in the outcome or the symptom. So changing the answer without addressing the factors would be wasted time and would propagate misunderstanding. So how do we address this wrong outcome or symptom? We go back and explain or demonstrate; if we have two apples and we add two more apples, how many apples do we have? As a parent we have now helped our child understand the factors that make up the result or the answer and by doing so we have changed our child's understanding and therefore changed the result.

How is this different than all of the results we experience in our day-to-day life that we do not like? If a smoker gets lung cancer is this much of a surprise? Smoking plus time equals a very high likelihood of disease, and cancer is certainly high on the list, but many others could have just as easily shown up. In this case, however, it was cancer first. The oncologist cuts, radiates and poisons in an attempt to save the person's life and due to wonderful new strides in technology, pharmacology and radiology, the rate of survival has risen dramatically. To follow the previous example above we have become incredibly skilled at turning the undesirable result, in this case cancer, into no cancer, or making the seven turn into a four, without the corresponding understanding of why cancer was created in the first place? I use smoking and cancer as an example we are all familiar with. However, I am here to tell you the majority of all diseases are created in this same way. For those of you reading these pages who were born before 1970 remember, the correlation between smoking and cancer were not even established. Can you imagine it has only been a few decades since someone asked the question and people started thinking, putting toxic chemicals into my lungs can cause a disease of my lungs? I predict in 50 or hopefully fewer years, people will read these words, and say "of course," how we live our daily life causes our diseases. It is all common sense. Sounds silly, doesn't it? Most of us have never considered that we cause most of the issues we experience in our life? We usually think it came from someone or somewhere else.

By no means should we diminish the need to address the outcomes or the diseases that are present in our experiences. However, as a physician whose aim is to prevent, I am challenging you to look at things from the position of cause rather than effect. Modern medicine in all its complexities is a perfect example that we can never address the cause by focusing on the symptom. Just like we can never find the error in our math equation by focusing on the incorrect answer, we must go back and look at the factors we used to create the outcome.

**GUILT HAS VALUE IN THE PROCESS OF CHANGE**

Often when people begin to embrace new understanding, and new perspectives their first response is guilt, i.e., I'm hopeless, I'm too far gone, I'm screwed up, I'm so bad. Although common, these feelings have little value in helping you create a new tomorrow. In fact, if your current perspectives continue, you will have no choice but to remain exactly where you are. We reference guilt now because if we do not understand its role in our life, it can have a largely debilitating effect on positive life changes. Guilt has a tendency to keep us stuck in a mode of negative self-assessment if we do not understand its purpose: A painful past lesson, which can be a valuable reminder in preventing us from doing something again. Our recognition of these old cause and effect experiences help guide us in a direction different than the choice we made in the past. Remember, "Change creates growth" is true for any part of your life, however the second part, which applies to guilt, is equally important: "acceptance creates peace." None of us can undo the wrong choices we have made in our life, or can undo the wrongs we have done to ourselves or others. Guilt is like poking an old wound every time you think of it, making yourself feel the pain and open the wound again. Remember what you learned from it but do not continually torture yourself. Self-torture is another form of stress, which holds you in a cycle of living the same life pattern, certainly NOT what we are going for. As we discussed above this does not mean we forget about the negative choices we have made. Learning from the past and regurgitating the pain is not the same thing. Learn and accept that you did your best at the time, and make a commitment to yourself that you do not desire to live that experience again. This recognition will stop the cycle that keeps many of us ruminating over and over about our past failings, and will allow what you will learn in the coming pages to move you forward in a positive new direction.

## THE FACTORS AFFECTING YOUR HEALTH

The variables of our daily life seem very complicated, when we ask ourselves, why am I overweight, why am I in constant pain, why do I have this disease condition or that. As illusive as it all seems, it is actually quite simple when you understand a few basic principals about nature, and for our discussion "The NATURE OF OUR BODY."

> **Resistance:** Resistance in life has potentially two outcomes. It can either create change or counter resistance (an opposing force that would be greater than, less than or equal to the resistance). Imagine the water in a river for a moment, if you observed either a large raging river of a small trickling brook you would notice whatever the water doesn't go over it goes around. If resistance is in the path of the water, the pressure builds at which point again, the water either pushes through the resistance or goes around. You will

notice also if there are no barriers the water flows effortlessly.

Now imagine, you place a dam anywhere along the water's path, the resistance of that dam must at all times exceed the pressure of the building water otherwise the dam will break. Consider how much force that dam must resist at all times. Now imagine if there was weakness anywhere in that structure. How would that impact the dam's ability to resist the pressure?

This analogy applies to our bodies too. We have a great ability to resist the forces of life, however, how much energy is required and at what point can our body and its systems no longer resist the forces? For everyone the amount of force before collapse may be different, but the forces that affect each one of us are the same. This is called STRESS.

Are the stressors in our daily life any different than the building pressure of the water on a dam? They come and we resist the small ones we handle but how much energy does this consume, how much resistance can we all tolerate? When big things come, loss of job, divorce, financial challenges, a death in the family, is that the breaking point? As we mentioned earlier for each of us it is different based upon our constitution and the adaptive mechanisms of coping we have adopted over our lifetimes, when we can no longer resist the pressures of life something will always give. For some this may be a nervous breakdown, depression and/or insomnia. For others it will be the alteration of physiology (how the body works), cancer, ulcers, glandular and hormonal imbalances, autoimmune diseases, fibromyalgia, lupus, rheumatoid arthritis. For others it may be back pain, muscle spasms, disc herniations, joint conditions, headaches or even numbness and tingling within the body.

When the resistance or stress can no longer be resisted by the body, breakdown MUST occur. In our modern day society we give these breakdowns specific names which indicate the particular area or system that has broken down. What confuses most people is the area of the body that has broken down is rarely the cause of the problem. Sounds confusing, doesn't it? Let me explain. If you break your leg from being hit by a car, you could say I HAVE A BROKEN LEG! This is true. However, if you are in the business of preventing broken legs, you would not be so concerned with legs, you would be much more concerned with the things that create large forces on the legs, like cars hitting them, or baseball bats being swung into them or sports that put undue stress on them. In the case of most modern disease to which we give complex, Latin based names, the disease is not the cause of the problem it is the name of the result. Like the broken leg, YES a lot of pain has resulted and one must deal with the RESULT, which would be the DISEASE that has a name, but if you are in the business of PREVENTING DISEASE you would most likely want to consider WHAT CAUSES that ORGAN or SYSTEM to BREAK DOWN. Our current medical system needs to be in existence to address these effects, i.e., the broken legs. However, the work that needs to be done so people can change their life, and create health must be focused in a different direction.

So where does that leave us? For the majority it is lost in the confusing details of diseases. Sadly that is what our institutions support. We do not have large conglomerates that teach people how they create their health conditions. Instead, our infrastructure supports beautiful palaces where we can go to address the emergency outcomes of our disease. In other words it is not easy finding answers in an ingrained system that has its primary focus on the results of our body's breakdown. How much different would the health of the world populations be if we examined and put our finances into reducing the stressors that create the breakdown in our body.

Never fear, **we have now found the purpose of this book**. There is good news, you do not need to find the needle in the haystack, because there is no needle to find, there is no Harvard graduate neurosurgeon, PhD, oncologist, gynecologist, podiatrist, proctologist, nephrologist, head of the biggest most prestigious hospital across, the oceans, on the top floor, of the golden palace in Dubai. There is no mystery. You have everything you need right now exactly where you are. Very anticlimactic isn't it? So if you don't need anything to get to the cause of your conditions how come you have the issues you have? The answer is simple, **"You have everything you need,**

**except the understanding of why you are getting the results you do not want."**

Like the child learning how to add, as described earlier, when understanding changes, outcomes change. The purpose of the pages ahead, are very simple….to build understanding and create new outcomes.

Many of you will disregard the remainder of this book because you are looking for someone or something to save you, and that is OK, it simply means that pain (whether it be physical or otherwise) from your current condition has not yet exceeded the perception of the pain that will result from change. For those of you who are ready to build an understanding this will absolutely change your life, you will find those seeds for change in the following chapters. One caveat before we proceed, the longer a condition or outcome has existed the more difficult it will be to reverse its effect. In other words, the longer a car goes without oil, the bigger the problem! There will come a time when the engine starts on fire and burns. Adding oil at this point has no value and does not offer the same solution it did early on. Many people have very serious and debilitating health conditions. What we will learn in the coming pages will no doubt furnish great improvements in all areas of your life and for your health. However, a person who is dying with lung cancer could certainly benefit from what you will learn in this book, yet he or she is at a state of great emergency that must be addressed. From the example above, the bigger the problem the fewer the options, and thus this should be a swift kick in the butt for all of us to do something now, before the possibility of being healthy is burnt to the ground. "We have the most power early on in the cause and effect cycle, the possibility of changing late in the cycle of disease still exists, however the effort becomes much, much greater and the results less gratifying."

For those of you who are in the early stages of any health condition, the course of your life can be directed to avoid the majority of the afflictions of our society. Your proactivity will furnish you great reward. For those of you with long patterns of symptoms and long lists of diagnosis, your life too can change course, however, more patience and more time will be required. Time and patience will be needed in direct proportion to the degree of your disease state. One of the most inspiring statements I give to my most desperate patients is simply this. "As long as you are alive you can improve, just like as long as you are alive you can get worse." The direction you take will be the one you choose.

### The "Origin" of Our Life Experiences

LET'S BEGIN

> Welcome to a new beginning. Before we go any further we must first look into why we experience the life that we currently live. Most of us ask why am I sick, why did this happen to me, or what did I do wrong to deserve this or that. Although these are common questions they actually bypass the biggest question that most of us are afraid to ask, which is: **How did I** create the circumstance that caused me to experience this or that? This means, what events accumulated to create the health experience you are living? The hard questions

are sometimes difficult to take, however it is essential to ask and eventually discover new answers if you truly want to change the outcomes. In this case it would be to exchange the experience of disease to one of health.

Lets first look at what drives our actions. We are all living our life based upon definitions we have either adopted from others or concluded from our own observations of life. These definitions are what drive our actions and of course lead the direction of our life. Whatever direction we are going creates our results. If these results are desirable to us we are happy; if they are not then we are unhappy. It's as simple as that, how the results are attained are the same in either case. We had a belief, that belief opened our mind to various reasonable possibilities based upon those beliefs. Our actions were then directed towards one or several of the reasonable possibilities that existed because of those beliefs and an outcome then occurred. Whether these steps were taken consciously or unconsciously is irrelevant. They were taken and in time a result occurred.

The above is the cycle of belief, it goes like this– we entertain thoughts of possibilities based upon or beliefs --we take actions based upon those possibilities – outcomes result, (effects of these choices). These choices may have taken many years to occur, however, it always works the same. So I ask you now, what are the outcomes you would like to change?

Exercise #1. Use a separate piece of paper and write down what you would like different. Perhaps you would like that chronic pain to go away, perhaps you would like to lose some weight or gain strength, or be done with that chronic fatigue, perhaps your would like to get out of debt, or have a better relationship with something or someone. Use this time to write down any component of your health or life that is not to your liking. As most of us know, we cannot possibly change anything that we are unaware of? Let's define what we would like to change.

Exercise #2. Now in a separate area below the above exercise, write down all the things in your life that are to your LIKING. Think of all the aspects of your life you are content with, that you enjoy, which make you happy. Make the list as long as possible and if you need more space, grab another piece of paper.

So your list on the left column at the top should have all the aspects in your life you are not that happy with, underneath that list is all the aspects that you are happy with. Now draw two columns from top to bottom to the right of your lists. Label the first column ACTIONS and label the second column BELIEFS. You have now just created a flow that will help you determine what actions and beliefs have helped create the things in your life that you like and those you do not like. OUTCOMES (what you like of dislike)----Actions---- Beliefs.

Now you will want to complete the next few columns, think about what actions could have contributed to bringing about the outcomes you do not like. For example, let's consider cancer as an outcome. What are the possible actions that could have contributed to this result? Perhaps one is a smoker? Perhaps one eats unhealthy processed food, perhaps one is exposed to regular doses of chemicals, or radiation from work or environment, maybe one takes medication to manage several other conditions, like pain medications, anti-inflammatories, perhaps one regularly applies chemical based products on to their skin, hair or nails. Look deeply at all the different possibilities that could have potentially contributed and accumulated to affect your body's inability to adapt and could possibly support the growth of cancer cells, or suppress your body's ability to destroy unhealthy cells.

Do not perform this exercise and feel bad about yourself, as this is not useful. Instead, look at your conditions as though you are not you. Be objective as though a friend has asked you to do this exercise to help them. Perform this activity as a scientist who is working to discover all the possible options that could contribute to a problem. When we look at our challenges from a new perspective we can cultivate a new awareness. Becoming aware of aspects that you had previously not acknowledged, allows possible solutions that we have previously not considered.

Now perform the same exercise for the outcomes you like or enjoy. What are the possible actions that could have contributed, for instance if you feel strong and healthy. Perhaps you have made choices to exercise regularly; maybe you avoid certain foods that are harmful, as an example. Maybe you have a great work environment, and you enjoy it, as an example of something you are happy with. Now what are the possible actions that have brought this about? Maybe you show up on time every day, you follow through with your work and complete tasks as expected, perhaps you are respectful to your co-workers and employer, or you go above and beyond the basic expectations to care for customers. Let's consider another example; perhaps you have a great relationship with your spouse, what possible actions could have contributed to this experience? This exercise is very important. The more detail, time and effort you put into discovering what contributed to your life's outcomes the more benefit to you. This exercise will help you look within and help you understand that most of what you experience you have allowed and supported through your actions. Yet the actions still are not the cause they are the movements and choices you made that were supported by your beliefs.

Let's, now look at the far right column, **BELIEFS**. As we look at the example of the disease cancer we listed a few possible actions that could accumulate over time to create the outcome of cell overgrowth or cancer. Now I ask you to entertain the idea that your beliefs could somehow make it possible to experience this sort of disease, stay with me a little longer. For instance, a belief that cancer runs in your family has the potential for a person to accept that cancer is a likely reality for them. Does this affect its potential of occurring? If you consider this objectively you would be bound to say yes. Let's look at a different subject. Imagine if you had a belief that you are poor, you have been poor, and your family has no money and barely gets by. Imagine this belief to you is part of who you are. Now let's imagine someone comes up to you and says you can have endless financial abundance, you do not need to be destitute and everyone has the same capacity for income as anyone else. Would you believe this statement? It is in fact absolutely true; however, your belief will keep your mind from accepting and allowing actions for its manifestation to occur. Because of your belief your openness to new possibilities to create income would not exist, if others offered opportunities, there would be a high likelihood that you would not accept them due to your self judgment of who and what you are, your habits would stay the same and of course your outcomes would stay the same. You have now again created the outcome you expected based upon your belief of whom and what you are and what you are able to have or accomplish.

Back to the cancer runs in my family belief. What are some of the possible actions one would entertain if this was a long-held belief? For most it would be outright acceptance, which as time goes by would influence the choices you make and the possibilities you entertain. For others it would be opposite, "I'm not going to let that affect me." Both cases and any response in between will change the outcomes or the possible actions one would participate in during their daily life. And of course each outcome would change based upon the overriding belief one holds. If the belief is supportive of the idea that your body is strong and capable and you have everything you need, and/or whatever you don't have will become available when you are open to it, versus my body is inherently flawed and susceptible to decay and disease and cancer is higher on the scale of probability. Whichever idea you subscribe to will result in different outcomes. We have all been around people who are very pessimistic. We have all been around people who are very optimistic. How do you feel around each person? Pessimism tends to suppress our energy level, while optimism tends to elevate our energy level. One makes you feel low, tired and fatigued, one makes you feel empowered, energized and in control. Did anything change but your mind in the moment? Imagine a lifetime around the pessimism versus and lifetime of the optimism; would your experience and your personal potential change? I believe if you look at it honestly you would have to agree it would.

You may have noticed that we have beliefs on all sorts of things in life. I am encouraging you to evaluate some of the aspects of your life, the aspects you enjoy and the aspects you would like to change. You will see your beliefs affect your actions, and your actions affect your experience. Some of you may deny this to be the case, of course that is just another belief, which would affect your outcomes. If the belief is we have no control over what we experience and life is a gamble, again your actions will support this, and your experience will be life is but a gamble. Funny how it works, isn't it?

> For the exercise you are working on above look into possible beliefs that could have driven your actions. You may find in your pondering that the results in your life that you do not desire tend to result from actions and beliefs that have a suppressive affect on your mind or your body. And the outcomes that you do desire tend to result from actions and beliefs that are supportive, positive and have uplifting effects on your mind or body.
>
> **EXAMPLE Worksheet**
>
> Outcomes you are not happy with
> Actions                          Beliefs
> -
> -
> -
> -
> -

-

-

Outcomes you are happy with
Actions                         Beliefs

-

-

-

-

-

-

-

So we have now identified the outcomes, diseases or
conditions we are unhappy with. Many of us have made
it this far before, which is great, but no change can
occur if we stop here. Outcomes did not originate the
problem you are experiencing. They are but a result of a
chain of events which created your current life
conditions, good and bad. More plainly, if your car
started on fire because you ran out of oil you would not
think that by putting out the fire you have corrected the
cause of the problem, which in this case is is a lack of oil
in your car. Just as if you found some medication to
reduce your symptom, you would clearly know the
cause has not been corrected. So the purpose of this
self-reflective exercise is to create a shift in your
perception. To look for cause rather than effect, a
foreign concept for most in a society that has been

engrained to expect immediate gratification, from self created symptoms.

Although this exercise seems a bit petty it is very important. Sadly, the majority of our world and unfortunately the majority of our health infrastructure spend its time looking at the outcomes and spending little time truly seeking the sources that creates our disease conditions.

The realm of beliefs can get messy, because most of us have never considered why we do what we do, we simply do it. So what we are looking at now is not just why we do what we do in and effort to change our life, but also asking ourselves, are we willing to input new beliefs, in an effort to change our lives? Are, we ready to slowly over time plant new seeds of thoughts, which in time can create new possibilities for life?

# 2

## Changing Beliefs

The first belief or seed we must modify is our definition of health. Most of us have never really asked ourselves "What Is health?" With no definition we then adopt the default belief from our parents, grandparents, media, symptom-based physicians or any other influences we have consciously or unconsciously allowed to influence us. What we have as a result is an operating system, or a belief that now becomes the infrastructure of all parts of life that relate to that subject of "health."

The overriding belief most of us have is, "Our body is inherently flawed"and therefore we expect problems to occur. As we age we expect more problems to occur because that is what we have observed with people as they get older. Therefore our belief of an imperfect body creates the expectation of problems which we observe become more and more frequent as we age until we finally die. We look around and see this happening and because we label ourselves realists we openly accept this to be true. Although there are many circumstances and people all around us that are living a different experience, we then consider them exceptions to the rule. We have created and label them as lucky, or perhaps if we are one of them we label ourselves as lucky, never aware of the possibility that our belief was part of the equation.

So a belief that disease is normal, and is expected, creates conditions that we do not like but expect. This idea results in so much undue suffering, and keeps the pharmacies hopping on every corner of every town and keeps the doctors of symptom management booked months in advance and our health insurance premiums continue to rise at the burden of misunderstanding. WOW. What if there is a different thought, would different possibilities become options? The answer of course is a resounding, YES!

What if our belief was that "Our body's natural state is health, its natural state is vitality, energy and efficiency" would that change the possible outcomes we experience? If we look around us we would have to agree that it would. With a new belief about our body's natural state we would stop accepting that illness, disease and symptoms are expected and normal, we would then ask ourselves different questions. Instead of questioning why is this happening to me or just accept that disease is something we must endure as we are busying ourselves looking for new symptom managers. We would instead ask ourselves the new questions. How did I make possible this disease process possible? How did my thoughts, words and actions influence my body's ability to maintain its natural state of health? How did I either consciously or unconsciously limit my body's capacity to heal? What have I done to create resistance to my systems that it now makes disease, dysfunction and symptoms a possible outcome?

Could we agree that if we believe we created resistance that now we would be able to entertain an entirely different realm of possibilities? At the beginning of this book we spoke about resistance and differences. Many people as they read the beginning of this book asked the questions. What does this have to do with health, what does the worlds social interactions between groups have to do with health? What does war between differing religious or government systems have to do with why I am sick or unhealthy? The answer is simple. It is everything, because resistance between people and groups creates conflicts, resistance in your body creates similar conflicts. Instead of calling it war or rebellion we call it disease, illness and symptoms.

Now imagine the possibilities of the paradigm shift, "our natural state of being is healthy, we create through long term resistance or stress, disease." So the question now becomes how do we create resistance rather than how do we manage disease? With this new understanding we can now empower ourselves with the mission of understanding. Understanding how we create barriers to our own experience of health and well being. How different would it be, instead of continuing our current dilemma of chasing our tail with the cycle of symptom, manage symptom, why is this happening to me, symptoms, manage symptom, why is this happening to me routine. To the let's deal with and remove the resistance we have created. Allowing us to replace ongoing stressors with the actions of reducing stress, thereby creating the environment to heal and support the body's natural and inherent desire to heal and to manifest health.

RESISTANCE creates STRESS. STRESS creates a protective response, the greater the stress the stronger the response, the longer the stress occurs the greater the influence on the actions of life, when balance can no longer be maintained something has to give.

Let's look again at our interaction with other people. If I push you, without thinking you will push back against me. Now if I am stronger than you, you will fall over or vice versa. I can only resist as much as my physical capacity will allow. If your capacity exceeds mine then I am overcome by the physical stress of you. Our conditioning, which has created our beliefs as mentioned above, has trained most of us to think you must meet resistance with resistance. Now let's consider a martial arts master, through his/her training they have developed an entirely different approach which creates different results. That approach is that you must not resist force with force, if you do there will never be any other option but the larger force wins (the big guy) and the smaller force loses (the little guy). It is a pretty cut and dry concept if that were the only option. However, a master martial artist has a different definition, which is you must flow with the forces that are directed at you and with this flowing you can redirect these forces which has little to do with strength and much more to do with awareness, skill and adaptability. This approach allows the variable of physical strength and size to become much less important for the purpose of conserving physical energy and by overcoming an opponent who is much larger.

This same understanding can apply to the cells of the body as it applies to stress (we will identify the various forms as we proceed), stress in its various forms creates resistance, like if you were pushing against me in the above example. My cell's capacities to resist these stresses are based upon what we can call my constitution. For instance, George Burns (the famous comedian) smoked his entire life and died at age 100. We could say his constitution to ward off the stress of smoking was better than a lot of other people, much like if my physical muscles are bigger than yours I could push you harder and for a longer period of time than you could me. This we can call our individual constitution to resist certain stressors.

Each person's body has various strengths and weaknesses, which increase or decrease their ability to resist life's strains. However, all stressors are the same. People often ask why did so and so get sick and I did not? We can understand why diseases appear in different forms when we understand that each person's strengths and/or weaknesses are different and therefore how diseases present themselves are based upon each individual's constitution or genetic predisposition. For simplicity let's define constitution as ones unique ability to resist various stressors. Some of us have greater abilities, some of us have less. No matter what our constitution, these stressors affect all of us to varied degrees no matter who we are.

The remainder of this book will not be based upon how to resist better or how to make you push back at life more. Rather, it will be on how to stop or reduce the creation of resistance or stress and allow the natural state of health in your body to flow. Much like the martial artist learns how to redirect and flow with the force of their opponent. We will learn how to remove the self-created resistance to health and in time undo the effects of resistance, which in time will create a greater experience of health.

THE ONE CAVEAT TO THE PREVIOUS PAGES

Many of you are saying this is all bologna, I have had this condition my entire life, parts of my body have been surgically altered, parts of my brain and nervous system are dead, there is no way that can be undone. Those of you thinking this are absolutely right, if your condition has gone to the point of surgery's removal of parts and pieces, destruction of neurologic tissue (nerves, brain, spinal cord) and permanent damage you CANNOT get to exactly where you want to go. If you want complete reversal of your condition this is highly unlikely, however, you are not doomed, to staying the same and worsening. By following the steps outlined in the coming pages, you WILL improve, but you may not get to exactly the state you would like to be. It's like a cavity in your tooth, the earlier you identify and correct the conditions causing the problem the better the outcome. Some of you have created enormous conditions of disease in your life. Full resolution for some of you may not be possible, however, no matter how big your problem is your body's natural state is health. So when we begin removing the causes it will always respond. How much it will respond will be related to how big the problem is and how long it has been there, but you can rest assured it will ALWAYS improve. What other options do we really have? Doing nothing guarantees more of the same, more disease, more pain, more suffering. Which option do you chose?

If you are alive, there are only two possibilities as it applies to your health: you will either get worse or better. We do have a choice in the matter. All this talk about beliefs and outcomes, stress and resistance is simply to expand your understanding. So that you can bring about the possibility that most of us have never entertained; can I make choices that will allow me to improve versus continue on my default course of worsening.

**Chapter Summary**

Health and disease are outcomes. Outcomes are results that have come from years of positive and negative influences on the body. These influences result in our body's ability or inability to resist the stress to its systems. Each individuals system has various constitutional or genetic strengths and weaknesses. These either protect us more than others or make us more susceptible than others to the action of resisting stresses. When the body can no longer resist the various forms of stress breakdown occurs. Depending on the type of breakdown that occurs, various diseases result. This is the disease creation cycle. Our current health systems deal primarily with resisting the outcomes or symptoms of disease. And is one of the major reasons as a nation and world we are spending more energy, time and money on health related issues and seeing chronic disease rising.

Healing can only occur by understanding this cycle and implementing a new mode of operation, by first changing definitions, then changing actions and in time changing outcomes. Finally, there is always the opportunity for change. However, the greater the destruction of the body systems, the lower the likelihood of complete reversal of any condition.

On the following pages we will help your "rescue yourself, from the affect of stress" so that you may create health.  Not by becoming better at resisting stress but rather by creating less stress to the body systems. When we reduce or eliminate stress or resistance the body's natural state of health will occur.

Which leads us to the next logical question, what is stress and how do we create less of it in an effort to experience better health?

# 3

## Stress and the Body

The first step to identifying resistance to your body's health is to understand that our body makes no differentiation of what your stress is. It just responds. Your body doesn't care if you lost your job; you can't pay the bills, are putting toxic chemicals into your body or filling your mind with negative, pessimistic or angry thoughts. It just responds.

These responses create a very physical outcome. For instance, if someone is holding a gun to your head, you could imagine you would feel a rush of adrenaline and you would be compelled to react in some way. This reaction can come in the form of a physical response, i.e., RUN, fight, kick or scream, or a physical response of NOT RUNNING. No matter what choice you would make a response occurs. Although they both look different to the observer, i.e., run or don't run, the internal effects are identical. Within your body chemicals would be released that would change your entire internal chemistry. Your body would suppress the immune system, to rally up efficient energy for one of your responses. Since your immune system protects you from microscopic invaders that can make you sick, your body in its wisdom would divert energy away from this system since there is a much greater eminent danger the time (gun to your head). Your body would then drastically reduce blood flow to most of your internal organs with the exception of the heart and would redirect that blood to the muscles of the body, to support the decision to run, fight or scream. In the brain chemicals would also be released, not just adrenaline from the kidneys, but inside your brain, chemicals that affect the opiate (opium like) receptors (sensors) would be released to numb pain receptors in case you get injured or shot. These chemicals will help keep the pain from stopping you from performing a life-changing action.

Since in this example your life is very much in danger your body will need quick energy, which for your muscles would be glucose (a type of sugar that gives your cells energy). Although energy could be attained from your fat storage, your body knows this is slow to happen so it makes sure to release chemicals to prevent you from using your energy from fat and only allows energy to be used from the blood stream. After this immediate form of energy runs out, the next quickest way to get energy is from the liver. In time this form of energy will also be exhausted and will need to use the next fastest source of quick energy, muscle tissue. The logical question would be why would the body take energy from the muscles instead of fat? Especially when the purpose of fat is to store energy and the purpose of muscle is to perform some form of movement. The answer is simple – efficiency. Remember in the example above someone has a gun to your head. Time is not a luxury you have, and muscle metabolism yields energy faster than fat, especially when the hormones of stress are floating around.

So where were we? The body's stress response, stress hormones up, blood flow to organs of building and repairing reduced, immune system suppressed, blood pressure high, to get blood to muscles fast, fat metabolism stopped and muscle breakdown for energy high. The perfect scenario for the moment, the perfect adaptive change to increase your likelihood of surviving the event of someone holding a gun to your head, but as we said earlier your body only has one response to stress, the only difference is the degree of the response. Now the scenario mentioned above is very dramatic and therefore the response is also more dramatic then it would be for a less strenuous event. However the mechanisms are the same regardless of the events. All that changes will be the degree of the response. So fat metabolism will stop or slow, muscle burning will be promoted, blood pressure will elevate, blood vessels will constrict, fat storage will be promoted and sleep will be disrupted. What would happen if this continued indefinitely?

Now imagine the gun to the head scenario again, invariably an end will occur. Either you get away or you are finished. Now let's imagine what happens if you got away. The stress hormones will reduce, your body will no longer feel threatened, blood will be redistributed to organs and systems that are necessary for repair, your immune system function will be restored, your blood pressure will drop, your blood vessels will relax and your body will push towards using fat stores for energy versus muscle. You will begin to repair, restore and rebuild from the stress you just endured.

**WHAT HAPPENS WHEN THE STRESS DOES NOT END?**

From the above scenario, most of you reading this could predict what would occur if the stressors do not come to an end. What happens if the equilibrium is not restored? Clearly blood pressure stays high, the immune system stays suppressed, and damage to your systems due to the inflammatory affects of the stress hormones on your cells would increase. Body mechanisms of repair would remain diverted, blood sugar imbalances become an immediate and constant battle for the pancreas (one of the blood sugar regulation organs) and risk of diseases rise. So how do we survive? Look around your neighborhoods, your hospitals, your work, your community. We are all experiencing what happens when this cycle does not stop. Name the top three life threatening diseases in our nation. Are we managing the stress effect?

**THE DISEASES OF MAN**

Is it that difficult to imagine why heart disease is the number one killer in the world? Or why in the year 1900, five percent of the population had high blood pressure whereas today over 30 percent have high blood pressure worldwide. Or why in 1980, 153 million cases of type II diabetes existed worldwide, yet today

347 million exist. We have more than doubled the occurrence of these very stress related conditions in just over 30 years.* What is to come of us?   (*Richard Johnson MD Nephrologist, University of Colorado Denver, National Geographic, August 2013)

When one has a general understanding of the stress response of the body, it does not take a doctorate degree to conclude that stress without end results in a very predictable disease creation patterns. Cancer, due to the continual immune suppression, heart disease and diabetes, due to the continual blood sugar balancing act, chronic inflammation due to the constant demands on the body without repair. What about the diseases associated with ongoing inflammation and immune suppression? Diseases like fibromyalgia, Systemic Lupus Erythematosus, Neurodegenerative disorders (Alzheimer's, MS, and Parkinson's) – they can all be linked back to the continual stress cycle, and the body's inability to maintain balance.

So what was the initial seed of this cycle? A belief or perception or reaction, I AM IN DANGER. In the above example it was a gun to your head. Thankfully for most of us this event will more than likely never occur. However, as we mentioned earlier whether an event is actually occurring or not is irrelevant, the perception of its occurrence is all that is required. The response when one really considers it has nothing to do with whether it is actually occurring and has everything to do with what you "think" is occurring which may or may not be the actual event. This should be very interesting to those of you reading these pages. Stress has more to do with perceptions of events than it does with the events themself. So where do our perception come from? You got it – OUR MINDS!

Stress Culprit #1 THE MIND, Ally or Enemy?

We have all heard the saying we get what we expect! If we expect success the outcome is generally successful and if the contrary occurs we consider this an unusual outcome. The same can be said for failure, if we expect a negative outcome we are rarely surprised when the opposite occurs. So for us to change our expectations we must look at our mind and more importantly our beliefs. These beliefs allow us to entertain what is and is not possible for us.

Mike Dooley, in his series Thoughts Become Things, writes that thoughts are the tail of the dog, the dog being our beliefs. So he contends that if we would like to discover our beliefs we need only pay attention to our thoughts, and in time this will lead us to our beliefs, which we can then evaluate. The logical question that most of us will then ask is, why would I do that, or why do I want to pay attention to my thoughts? The simple answer of course is you don't HAVE TO, but if you WANT TO, an opportunity for change becomes possible. Evaluating what makes up your choices and expectations will uncover some of the seeds that create the events in your life. This applies to the elements in your life you are fully content and those you are not. Many people have simply given up and become indifferent because they feel they never achieve the health or well being they desire. I hope you are not one of those, because once you understand the power of your beliefs and your mind you can truly get to the answer to the question "Why is my life the way it is, and how do I change it?" Of course only you know if you truly are ready to look, learn and make incremental changes, no matter where you are it all starts one step at a time first in the mind.

So, let's go back to thoughts. What drives the never ending flow in your head, what drives your expectations, your choices and invariably the outcomes you have experienced in life? If you read the beginning pages of this book you would be correct by saying "beliefs." Beliefs are your assessments of the world. Regardless of how correct they are or are not leads to your choices.

I hear this frequently with patients, "I'm old, this is what happens," "It's genetic," "I've always been heavy," "Everyone in my family has high blood pressure," "All of my family gets cancer" or "I will never get better." Ask yourself what are your thoughts around the challenges in your life, whether it is health, finances or any other topic? I believe if you look hard enough you will find a dominant thought on the topic and it's very likely some variation of the examples above.

Now, let's think about what a limiting belief like the examples above can do in our lives. Most of us consider these thoughts as absolute truths because of our experience, and no doubt we all have our reasons for believing what we do. However, looking around you, why do others have different experiences in their life? If everyone had the same belief system as you, believe it or not most people's lives would look very similar to yours. If for example everyone believed there is not enough of something, then how could anyone have abundance in anything, if YOUR or MY TRUTHS are the be all end all, nothing would have the opportunity to be any different then the way it is right now, based upon your current idea of what is true and what is not......UNLESS we change our minds, then and only then can different outcomes be possible.

This leads to the next logical question. If someone is or has something we want, we must ask ourselves, what idea or truth does that person have about this topic that we do not? This goes also for ourselves, if a friend says, "How are you so healthy, why am I so unhealthy?" You must ask yourself the question, what belief do I hold about health that is different from my friend? Whether you know what it is or not, you most certainly hold a different set of beliefs and perceptions than your unhealthy friend. This goes for everything, so for every person in the world we have some common personal truths and we have individual truths. So you ask which truth is the "RIGHT"? The answer of course is "all of them"! However, if you are not happy with your current experience you need to change "YOUR TRUTH, OR PERSONAL BELIEF" otherwise change cannot occur.

If you have ever watched the popular television show "The Biggest Loser" you see this in action. When a new contestant begins their process they have a set of beliefs about who they are, what they have done and what they are capable of. They spend the next several months in solitary confinement with a group of trainers, dieticians and psychologists who literally remove all the distractions from their life and over the course of many months reprogram the person belief system as it applies to health, weight, potential and capacity. Of course they also exercise, change their diet and surround themselves with new habits. These are all progressive steps which started with changing what they believed was possible for them. As a reminder, creation of anything first begins with thoughts, then words and finally action. In the reality show they address all components and what happens? If that person allows it to happen, the mind begins to change, habits begin to change, and finally the body begins to change. The success or failure of the contestants is based upon how much that person's entire system of operation is altered.

People say if they had a chef cooking their meals and a trainer pushing them to exercise they would get those results too. For the short term that may happen, but long term this cannot happen. The success of the contestants is based upon their personal desire to be different. The strength of their desire allows them to hold themselves in an environment that is incredibly foreign, and in time their beliefs about themselves changes and thus new possibilities become a reality. Their actions change and of course in time their body changes. The stronger the persons desire and the speed at which their beliefs change will determine the speed and degree of the physical change. If it was simply about a trainer and a chef, the purchase of these people's videos should be enough to create lasting transformation. What most people don't understand is that the belief transformation is the hidden secret of lasting change and this starts in the mind.

We see this similar phenomenon with people who have financial problems who win the lottery. Statistically the less money a lottery winner started out with the faster they will lose the money they have won. If you look at the long-term wealth of lottery winners, the majority of the winners are broke after just a few years. How can someone lose MILLIONS of dollars in just a matter of a few years? If you understand how the mind works, it makes perfect sense. Having money has little to do with the physical presence of money in your life. It has mostly to do with your beliefs and thoughts around the topic of money. For instance, if a person has deep seeded beliefs that money is hard to come by, that shortages are a normal part of existence or that whatever you have will always runs out, can you imagine how that would impact your decisions and choices if someone dumped a huge pot of cash in your lap? So, yes, these people get a large wad of money, however their beliefs which affect their actions have not changed. Invariably their circumstances in time HAVE TO go back to what their beliefs and actions support, which in this case would be running out of money again. Does this mean we are doomed? Of course not! If you are aware of the effects the mind has on our life. Remember again, the mind opens or closes the door to the possibilities that exist for you. Artificially changing our surroundings does not change our mind. Like the person who magically receives millions of dollars, or by getting plastic surgery to make our outer body look different or taking some medication to force our body to perform differently so our blood tests looks different. Change can only occur through understanding the roots causes of seeds of our conditions, the roots being STRESS. And the first stress we must understand is the stress we create in our mind.

**STRESS AND AGING**

My personal belief is that aging is a wonderful enriching progression. I tell my patients every day that life is like a great bottle of red wine. It just gets better with age. Most of my patients are quick to disregard this belief of mine, they laugh and say, "You're so young just you wait," or they simply laugh it off. Perform some of you own experiments, listen to others. Hear what they say and then from what you know of them determine if their life is an example of their statements. This is very easy to do with others, as you become more observant of others, look at yourself. Of course people's views on money are a great way to understand the belief/outcome relationship. Talk to people who have a lot of money, talk to those who do not, talk to the people who have the level of health you desire, talk to people who suffer from chronic conditions, become aware of the difference. I have observed that if you listen you will find there is no difference between what people are saying and what they are experiencing.

## How the Mind and our Beliefs create possible outcomes and possible choices

If I was to say you have two choices, black or white, and you had to choose which would you pick? For this example there is no right or wrong, just two choices. Each one will have a different event that precedes the choice. Every day in our own head we establish our choice of possibilities. These are based for the most part on our beliefs. If I had a belief that I will always be fat, the only choice I have given myself is the "I will always be fat" choice. The details of this can be confusing and complicated but for our purposes there is no other choice available because your belief has made only one option available….fat. If this is now the only option you allow you cannot even entertain the possibility of thin. Do you truly believe any sort of weight loss action, or lifestyle change that supports thin will exist? That being said what other options are there? You got it, there are no other options. So if a person who truly wants to change their body must work first on changing their mind about their body.

Have you ever wondered why the weight loss industry is a billion dollar and rising industry with a less than one percent success rate? Think about that, out of 100 people, one person successfully keeps the weight off indefinitely. What's different about them, you ask? By accident or by unconscious choice during their process they had a shift in their beliefs of who they are and the possibilities that exist for them, this opened an entirely new set of options, either by conscious choice or by accident. Either way a shift in the mind occurred that supported a new operating system as it applied to the habits which supported weight loss.

Instead of I will always be fat, their mind shifted to I can be and I am healthy. From that new set of beliefs new options became possible for them, as new choices were made and positive outcomes over time occurred, their thoughts and beliefs strengthened. With the strengthening thoughts and positive experiences to support these thoughts their beliefs became more ingrained and the possibility of lasting change became a greater and greater "reasonable" possibility. This in time led to a new reality, a different physical body.

You cannot change the problem by working on the symptom.

We see this every day in medicine, here take this pain medication, this antidepressant should help, but do any of them truly resolve the issues? We are of course, NOT discrediting the need for medications in our society to aid in the support of helping our symptoms. However, symptoms are not the problem, as annoying and frustrating as they can be, they are the symptoms. The oil light in your car is a symptom of no oil, a fire in your house could be as symptom of a bad electrical connection. Yes oftentimes like with a house fire you absolutely must put out the symptoms, especially when it compromises your entire home, but you can't get to the source through the symptom. In your car you would have to go under the hood, not lament over the oil light.

So why then are chronic pain, obesity, depression and many other conditions growing out of control? Requiring now the majority of Americans, adults and children, to take daily medication to suppress and manage the symptoms. I am sure you have figured it out. We have forgotten that symptoms are not the problem. We have accepted (another limiting belief) that they the symptoms are part of normal. Of course most of our medical profession has that similar belief. So you have a lot of very intelligent people in very large glass buildings holding this same belief and strengthening it, just like those who once believed the world was flat. By all means we come by it honestly and here we are again, experiencing the same thing over and over again, yearning for a new discovery, a new procedure or a new drug to "save us" from our self-created misery. We wish for different outcomes, yet sabotage ourselves simply because we do not allow the possibility of something different. Because as you know, "this condition or that is incurable, my doctor told me so."

Have you ever marveled at the fact of your conception? I'm not talking about the moment of your parents' connection, silly... remember this is a family book ☺. Two cells came together. Within those cells, the addition of the safe environment of your mother's womb, the nutrition provided by your mother and the instruction housed within your genetic code, "YOU" were created. Let that sink in for a moment.  All that was required to create you was two cells, instructions from within those cells (genetic code), nutrients and a safe supportive environment. When patients fear that they cannot improve, I remind them that within their body all that is necessary to improve exist when the environment is supportive.

Now let's mess around with the equation and see what happens. Remember Thalidomide, the morning sickness drug taken in the 1950s and 1960s? What happens when you introduce a foreign chemical into the mix of the very simple equation above? In the case of Thalidomide we saw over 10,000 "reported" cases of birth defects resulting from a drug "interfering" with the development of the growing fetus.

Do our medications help or hurt? We know they aid symptoms or change blood results and they can certainly save a life when a life is very close to ending, yet do medications truly help the body get healthy? I wish we could say they do, however in most cases, the long term effects actually weaken the body and create more stress to the body systems.

Pain is a symptom, obesity is a symptom, depression is a symptom, high blood pressure is a symptom, Parkinson's disease is a symptom, Alzheimer's disease is a symptom, cancer is a symptom, and death is a symptom. So what in heaven's name is the problem???

I think you know the answer! Stress!! It comes in three general forms with many sub-forms, but when it's all said and done there are only three. The first type of stress we have been discussing for some time now, mental stress, the resistance we create in ourselves from our thoughts, our beliefs, our fears and insecurities. These thoughts, no matter what form they take, create our words and actions. These thoughts again, no matter how they were created, either establish the environment of rest, rejuvenation and healing within our cellular environment of our bodies or create the environment of stress, anxiety and resistance within our cellular environment. The second is chemical and/or nutritional, the elements we put into our body either through food, chemical exposure and air. The third is physical, resulting from the demands of life, injuries, imbalances and physical forces.

As we discussed above the mind is the seed of all actions. For example if you need to go to the bathroom, you first acknowledge, my bladder is full. Then you formulate either verbally or without words in your mind, "I need to take a pee," and then you walk to the restroom and facilitate the action. Every action in our life follows the same process. Thought----word (verbal or non verbal)---deed (action).

From the mind thoughts are created, thoughts are generally based upon your belief system that was either established by you or in combination, you, your family, other people, your culture, and any other circumstances and events which influenced you. As we said before, the trueness of your beliefs is irrelevant. What is relevant is IF it is true for you. That is all that matters. Whatever is true for you opens various possibilities for you in your mind. If your beliefs hold the high probability of a positive outcome the likelihood of a positive outcome is very high. If the probability in your mind for a negative outcome is high then of course the likelihood of a negative outcome is high.

So what is the first stressor of the mind? Your beliefs! As we discussed above, these create your thoughts of likely possibilities in your life, so then the first step to becoming healthy has little to do with "doing" anything. It has first to do with evaluating your "being" which means those unconscious "beliefs" which run your life.

EXERCISE: DISCOVERING THE MIND

For the next week as you go about your daily life pay attention to yourself and the people around you. Practice the technique longtime author and speaker Dr. Wayne Dyer calls, "Thinking about, what you are thinking about." Dr. Dyer says that most of us have a runaway mind, that few of us ever have any idea what we are thinking about, and furthermore even less of us are aware that we can gain control of our thoughts, rather than letting our thoughts control us. How we begin is simple. Pay attention to yourself. What are you thinking about when you get irritated, when you get stuck in traffic, when you feel the need to eat a whole pint of Ben and Jerry's, when that chronic pain won't go away, when you feel like you are having a nervous breakdown, when you get angry, annoyed or uptight. On the flip side, what are you thinking about when you are happy, when you feel optimistic, when you are encouraging yourself or others? Start paying attention. If you commit to doing this as much as you can you will absolutely see a pattern.

Start by observing others. As the Bible verse goes, it is very easy to see the speck in your friend's eye, and much more difficult to see the mud in your own. As you observe, especially as it applies to the things in your life you are not happy with, you will see a pattern. From this pattern you then have a choice you did not previously have, the choice to choose a different thought. In time and with practice this will allow a different action or outcome.

This of course is the entire goal of affirmations and the many books by authors like Lois Hay, and others, the goal with these processes is to start with an encouraging uplifting statement and continually tell yourself something that is positive. The goal being in time that you start to believe it and when this occurs, your thoughts, choices and actions then become different. These books are based on the idea that we are impressioned by what we hear. Like a child our beliefs are established by the words we heard growing up by the people who influenced us. This applies to children as well as adults. However, the main difference with you and I, adults, reading this book, we now have self-awareness and can consciously make new choices. This practice of putting in new thoughts will ensure different outcomes then the ones we unconsciously developed as children. With new thoughts we now have choices, whereas when we were children we did not. How liberating it is to know you have the opportunity to change something you do not like in your life.

Once you pay attention to what you are thinking about, patterns will start to emerge. After several weeks you will begin to observe aspects of yourself you like and want to keep, and aspects perhaps that could be changed for your benefit.

Since this book is about creating the physical status of health to prevent disease, stop or reverse disease or just be proactive, pay special attention to your thoughts around health, about disease, about fitness, and about diet. Look to see what judgments you hold about yourself or others around these topics. My observation is if you give yourself enough time, and are honest you will run into what the author Mike Dooley calls "limiting beliefs," these are beliefs that put barriers up that prevent you from attaining something. A good example of a limiting belief to help you understand would be a person who wants to play basketball, however he "believes" he's too short. This belief of course has no real validity, but the person saying it limits their ability to play basketball because he has a belief that he must be of a certain height to play.

Imagine if you had a belief that you are destined for a chronic disease because your family has some condition, or you will always be heavy because you have always been heavy, as though it is not "possible" for you to reduce your weight. This too is a limiting belief.

There are many others, pay attention and see what you find. There is no doubt if you are honest and consistent you will observe some limiting beliefs that probably are not helping you get where you say you want to go.

## NOW HOW DO YOU CHANGE THOSE LIMITING BELIEFS?

Once you find them, then what? You got it, change them! Of course a little easier said then done, but what do you really have to lose?  So, how do you go about changing a belief? You replace it, with something that would be believable to you. THIS IS IMPORTANT. If I was obese and believed I could never lose a pound, and then someone asked me to imagine myself at a healthy weight, doing all the things healthy fit people do at the drop of a hat, this wouldn't be that believable to me. However, perhaps there is a more believable first step, for instance maybe you could imagine yourself being 10lbs less and getting out of a chair more easily. That approach seems believable if a person has had a lifetime of being obese.

Once you have become comfortable with your new believable belief then of course you can expand it further over time. I call this "MIND THERAPY." This mind therapy will build. Here's how it goes. You start believing you can lose 10lbs and move easier, keep reminding yourself of this very reasonable goal, in time you begin ACTING differently perhaps you eat a little less each time you eat, then perhaps instead of sitting for many hours you decide to get up more often, perhaps instead of drinking soda, you chose water. All these little changes from simply "deciding" to believe something different, there's another SECRET, there is no end to the changes that are possible for you. Guess what happens after you lose 10lbs and move more easily, YEP, you expand your belief further, you can now entertain a larger realm of possibilities. Now perhaps you believe that you would be capable of losing 40lbs, and walking two miles at a time. WOW, an impossibility prior to your first belief, but as you progress you will be reprogramming you mind, thus the term "Mind Therapy."

Remember when you hold a thought in your mind long enough you begin to accept it. If you want to experience quick changes in your life you must plant a new belief that is believable to you, and like a plant, water it with your attention and energy and it will grow.

If you have ever planted a garden you know that seeds and soil are only part of the equation of producing a bountiful harvest. With mind therapy, you must acknowledge your seeds of the past. Planting new seeds (thoughts/goals, etc.) that you can accept will create positive steps in the direction towards the changes that you are seeking. Planting the new idea in the soil of your open mind will allow it to begin the growing process. This isn't the whole story as it applies to gardening or changing your life. You also have other seeds you have planted, from the past or just by accident, like weeds in the garden these are competing for space in your mind and will impact the ability of your new vulnerable beliefs to grow. It is no surprise WHY most people rarely make long-term changes. They have never understood that new ideas, new beliefs and new truths become suffocated by the beliefs that are already established.

When I go on vacation and leave my garden unattended, in just a few short days may garden is overgrown with weeds. When I return I must make a great deal of effort to get my garden back in order. Our mind is so similar, when we stop being conscious or self-aware, our old patterns which are ingrained quickly overgrow. This becomes very frustrating to a person who desires change, and to most it dissolves their resolutions to continue. They feel overwhelmed, ineffective and defeated. These are expected outcomes if you do not understand the mind. I choose to plant a garden because I want the fruit it will bear. I also know when I take a vacation my garden will become overgrown, which is expected, so I will not be surprised when I get home and the weeds are high. I will know there will be more work to do because I have not tended to the weeds. Knowing that your beliefs of the past can take over if left unattended can free you from anxiety and guilt and keep you from reverting back to your old ways of thinking. The simple solutions: get back into the habit of supporting your new idea, thoughts or goals; water these positive changes with supportive information that you observe in others and yourself; shine the light on growing new perspectives by surrounding yourself with people who themselves are on a path of positive change. The birth of anything, such as an idea or a child, is messy and very labor intensive, states author MaryAnn Williamson. However, creation requires a great deal of initial effort and great faith, but once established much less effort is required.

If you desire to reduce self-created mental stress, it will be imperative to understand and apply the mind therapy process above. Remember, the majority of the good and bad in your life are created based upon the process of thoughts, words and actions. The only difference is that now YOU can begin choosing what seeds or thoughts you are planting. Choosing the thoughts and beliefs that help you, and denying energy and thought to those that harm your progression is a proactive process and gives you a CHOICE for change.

The exciting thing about "YOUR BELIEFS AND YOUR TRUTHS" is that they are changeable, all of them. Of course you would not want to change them all, just the ones that prevent you from creating the healthier version of yourself.

Exercises: POSSIBLE NEW THOUGHTS that can reduce your mental stress and change your life.

1. Everything works out for the best.
2. People are inherently good, with a few exceptions.
3. I am capable of achieving the life and environment I desire.
4. I am trustworthy.
5. Good things come to me, are available to me and are available to everyone else, whether they think so or not.
6. I am responsible for "ME," others are responsible for themselves, with a few exceptions, i.e., underage children, the physically or mentally handicapped.
7. I have the power to change what I do not like and to create what I desire. This will take time and persistence. The more consistent I am the quicker the changes I will see.
8. You can have all the money you desire, if your beliefs about money support abundance.
9. There is no shortage of resources; there is enough for everyone.
10. Competition does not exist unless you think it does.
11. No one is holding you back, even if it feels that way.
12. I am blessed.
13. My past does not need to define my future, unless I want it to! I can choose!

14. Everything that I see and hear has two different perspectives, a positive perspective and a negative. Which one I choose will determine my future. Choosing the positive perspective increases my optimism, my confidence and my power. The negative perspective increases my negativity, erodes confidence and supports the victim mentality.

15. Everything changes, nothing ever remains static and unless you are expending large amounts of energy to keep it static, this cannot succeed indefinitely. Accepting change will give you peace, adaptability and creates faith in the higher order of things.

16. I can choose what I want to see. Others can choose what they want to see also. If I do not like what I see I have choices.

17. Others have shaped me, however I get to define me, and chose the direction of my life moving forward.

18. Blame is a choice to give away your power. I chose responsibility. If I am responsible I can make the changes I desire. If I blame others I have given them the power to change me.

19. Acceptance acknowledges that things have happened, good or bad, but how they affect us is our choice. I choose a new and different perspective that helps me.

20. Each day offers new possibilities for positive change.

21. Realism is a focus on negativity and problems and is only one side of any perspective.
22. Optimism is not denial. It is a choice to focus on solutions rather than problems, the opposite of a realist and a pessimist. It is one side of a perspective and I choose positive.
23. It takes time, patience, persistence and practice to reprogram your mind.
24. I have created momentum in my life; new ways of living need time and energy to create momentum in a different direction. I have patience and persistence.
25. I took a lifetime to get me where I am. It will take some time to get me to a different point.

---

Pay attention to your responses as you read this list, one by one contemplate and consider each statement. Do you adamantly resist any one or several of them? Do you accept and support any? This list of course is a simple example of a few of the more positive, encouraging and supportive beliefs that one may have. If we consider our beliefs like software on the computer of our mind, we come to understand that our software can be altered by the programmer, YOU! If you would like to improve your operating system you need simply to begin reprogramming.

As you go thru your day, begin observing. Think about what you are thinking about. This is your first step in reprogramming, which is the first step in mind therapy. I encourage people to write some of their dominant thoughts down. The easiest way to discover your dominant thoughts is to observe your feelings. What makes you really irritated, what makes you really happy, what are some of the things that annoy you about yourself and others? Chances are you have a conflicting belief or beliefs that someone or something is challenging when you get irritated. Your reaction - happy, sad, angry or otherwise - is your mind's way of accepting or rejecting what you have heard or experienced. Write it down. Chances are there is some PROGRAMMING that is influencing your emotions. This programming is exactly what we are working on finding. From there we can keep it if we are happy with our response or look to change it if we are not.

Eckhart Tolle, in his books *The New Earth* and *The Power of Now*, calls these negative experiences, "The Pain Body," meaning that when something or someone makes you angry they are touching a mental wound, much like someone sticking their finger in a cut. This experience causes you emotional pain and suffering, and of course creates a response. If you have an experience that touches a painful belief, or reminds you of emotional pain, this will cause a reaction too. You will get angry, fight, withdraw or react in a myriad of different protective responses. Mr. Tolle writes that this creates much of our personal suffering and the majority of our conflicts, both on a personal level and a group level, all creating stress to the body's systems.

So what is the purpose of all this, what value does any of this serve? The answer of course, to build PERSONAL understanding, so you can create less self-induced stress, less pain, more proactive behavior, less reactive behavior, more joy and of course create health in your body; rather than an environment which strains our systems and allows diseases the opportunity to occur. Health in our body starts with PEACE, ACCEPTANCE AND UNDERSTANDING IN YOUR MIND.

Stress in the mind creates stress in the body. Stress in the body over long periods creates resistance to the systems. This reduces efficiency, reduces healing and is one of the three components of stress that break down our systems and compromises our health!

# 4

---

# We Are What We Think and We Are Also What We Eat

---

We have all heard the saying, "We are what we eat." But have you ever really thought about what that means? We discussed earlier that there are three major forms of self-created stress causing resistance to our natural state of health: Mental/Emotional, Nutritional/Chemical and Physical/Structural. So now the question is raised, what do food and other chemical components have to do with stress?

This is a question that few have ever pondered and fewer still have considered. How what we eat today builds our body for tomorrow? It has been said if you are wondering what tomorrow will look like, look at what you are eating, thinking and doing today. There is no better example than the example of what we put in our body, either through our mouth, our lungs or our skin.

So what we look and feel like today is a direct outcome of our many, many yesterdays. Of course we cannot change our yesterdays (for most this leaves them paralyzed in guilt, remorse and regret). However, we can certainly change our todays, all for the purpose of having a more desirable tomorrow. Sound complicated? It's not, when you really consider it. We mentioned earlier that our thoughts direct our life, which direct our words, which finally direct our actions. Is what we consciously expose ourselves to, either through our mouth, our lungs and our skin, just another action? Remember also, unawareness of how things affect us still creates a response in our body, whether we know it or not. That is why before any changes are made in the body and in our health it must start in the mind.

If I "tell" someone NOT to do something without knowing why, compliance by that person would only hold to the degree they BELIEVE I have AUTHORITY OVER THEM. Compliance to do what I demanded would be limited, if it was performed at all. If you did what I told you to it would not have occurred willingly, thus whenever someone with MORE perceived authority comes along the activity would be abandoned. However, if I "teach" someone a perspective or understanding that they have never known or considered, this person now has the understanding to make choices based upon a new set of criteria and thus action can be self motivated by understanding. This is called empowerment, giving YOU the perspective necessary to make new choices. Perception and understanding changes choices and opportunities. Our food consumption patterns are a wonderful example of this process.

What better place to see the dynamic of misguiding the uninformed than in our food industry? Natural flavorings, no calories, no fat, cholesterol-free, etc.; Our lack of understanding of the basic fundamentals of the body have allowed us all to be manipulated by professional looking ads, by labeling or by celebrity endorsement. Our goal here is to give you the basics of your body, and how we can all stop killing ourselves one forkful at a time, one lotion pump at a time and one spray of our countertop at a time. Sound dramatic? Let's see!

WE ARE WHAT WE EAT?

Let's look at the phrase "We are what we eat." Where does what we put in our mouth go? As we know, but perhaps haven't thought about, everything we consume either builds us, damages us or in a few rare occasions is neutral in its effect on our bodies. One thing we must NEVER forget is that "EVERYTHING" has some effect on our body and that's OK, if the majority of those things are supportive to its systems, its functions and your health. If they are not then it is bad news for us.

So, what happens with the food we consume? Let's take a look!

Before we get into the specifics of how our foods and what we are exposed to affect our body it will be important to get a basic understanding of the GI, or gastrointestinal tract (stomach, intestinal tract, bowels etc.), for when a basic knowledge is established the understanding of the downfalls we create become self evident, and new choices become common sense.

Your breakfast this morning started in your mouth. From there it is broken down mechanically, via your teeth. Your food was mixed together with saliva, which contains a few enzymes (body produced chemicals that help chemically break down food), where it is then swallowed and travels to your stomach. In the stomach, acid (yes, acid is necessary, contrary to the belief stomach acidity causes indigestion and needs to be neutralized; more on this later) is produced by the cells in the stomach. The purpose is to begin breaking down proteins. Proteins cannot be broken down and utilized in our bodies unless this acid is present and in adequate amounts. The stomach acid aids in the preparation of essential mineral absorption and ionization, especially calcium, magnesium and potassium. Preparation and absorption of vitamin B12 (the only be vitamin that requires a special protein found only in the stomach, called intrinsic factor) occurs also, which is essential for all tissue building and proper blood cell production. This is the only place this special vitamin can be absorbed and is only found in animal-based proteins.

Remember also that our body is primarily made up of proteins, fats and co-factors that come from vitamins and minerals. Replacement of these proteins, minerals and vitamins are absolutely dependent on the function of the stomach. If the stomach is not working or has been stalled by the use of medication, you will not get what you need to build and replenish your body's building supplies. In time, disease will always result.

From the stomach, the acidified partially broken down food now initiates the function of the small intestine. Its purpose is to further break down the food from the stomach, with the help of enzymes, chemicals that break protein, fat and carbohydrates into components that can be absorbed into the blood stream. Like the stomach, all steps depend on the previous to accomplish its task. When the nutrients from food, either can't be absorbed or are absorbed or broken down incompletely issues can occur, contributing to everything from gas/bloating and irritable bowel syndrome to chronic allergies.

The small intestine's purpose then is to break carbohydrates into sugar, fats into fatty acids with the aide of the gallbladder and liver and proteins which will be broken into smaller parts called amino acids. From there the rest of the 20-plus feet of intestines are designed to absorb these broken down carbohydrates, fats, protein and water, with the aid of various forms of fiber and helpful bacteria. Finally, it will expel the remnants of what the body could not break down and use, and any toxins that could be dumped into the intestinal track from other organ systems along the way.

Now we know the generalities of the GI tract, let's now look into what happens with the broken down food components are absorbed into the blood stream. In the blood stream most will go to the liver to be processed.

In the blood stream you not only have what you need - amino acids (protein), fatty acids and sugars, you also have what comes along with our food at various levels of the digestive process. For simplicity we will call them toxins of any sort, anything that your body does not need or cannot use. These toxins can be from colorants that were in the food you ate, hydrogenated or chemically manipulated fats, medications, foods that were not broken down properly, pesticides, preservatives, chlorine or hormones, just to name a few. These are all things that are not needed and must be stored, neutralized or expelled, all requiring the use of your body's energy and resources.

In the liver the blood stream processing occurs. Like a very efficient factory, useable items are used and dispersed, surplus items are stored for later use, damaging items are neutralized as best as possible by the liver, with the attempt of either expelling them, via the urine, or dumping back into the large intestine with the intent of being eliminated, or through other organs like the lymph system and sweat glands. Each organ will do its best to remove the damaging elements in an effort of protection and self-preservation. If these elements cannot be removed then the body will find a way to store these toxins.

It is a wonderful system that is designed to work and to be efficient "IF" balance can be maintained. However, what happens when balance cannot be maintained?

You got it, stress is created, which is a response to this imbalance. Of course, short-term stress is part of the wax and wane of life but what happens if balance cannot be regained? You see it in other areas of your life – a downward spiral begins. Large amounts of your body's energies are then used to try to protect your systems from the effects of these imbalances and diseases then begin to manifest.

THE TRILOGY OF DISEASE from Chemical/Nutritional Imbalance:

- Stress/Resistance from surplus
- Stress/Resistance from deficiency
- Stress/Resistance from toxicity

Above are the three main stressors we create from what we put into our body from eating, drinking, breathing or absorbing. Let's now look into how this occurs and then most importantly, how we can begin shifting to a state of less resistance and stress in an attempt to improve our health balance.

Surplus (too much), deficiency (too little) and toxicity (unwanted and damaging) stress is very evident in today's society. Take a look around. We spoke early on about sugar and the problems associated with such. Have you noticed our children? Take a look at the average fifth grade class. What do you see:  Obesity, illness, a rising use of medication for symptom management? Lack of awareness and lack of understanding, as well as toxic food and environments has caused an explosion of what could be called the trilogy of death (surplus, deficiency and toxicity) in action. The culprit can be easily identified. It is a lack of awareness, low food quality and lack of awareness of the basic fundamentals of anatomy. There is a funny saying that can be applied to the body. The saying goes you don't have to know how to build a cell phone to use it, however you do need to know a few fundamentals to be able to get the benefit of using it. You do not need to be a master of nutrition, biochemistry, neurology, anatomy etc., to use your body in a healthy manner, but you must grasp a few fundamentals to help you use it. If you don't know these fundamentals, the misuse will result in disease.

Now imagine we have low quality, high calorie foods from simple carbohydrates (processed grains, processed vegetable fats) and toxic food going into the body on a consistent basis. This food has very little nutritional or healing value yet it has a great deal of simple energy and calories. Once in the body, these unnecessary calories are quickly converted into fat for storage, sugars/carbohydrates are turned into triglycerides or fat, or if it is a fat it will be stored directly. A big misunderstanding amongst the world is the belief that sugar is not turned into fat. This created the fat-free craze of the 1990s. This generation stopped eating fat, everyone increased sugar consumption and got fat faster, while creating an even greater rate of heart disease and diabetes, all from the misunderstanding of physiology and strategic marketing.

Remember, nutritionally deficient foods do not contain the co-factors necessary for their processing. Therefore, the body will now have to pull out of storage vitamins, minerals and co-factors for the metabolism and processing of this food. The low quality food you now put into your body has created two forms of stress. 1. It has added energy surplus, which needs to be processed stored and maintained and 2. It has stolen from your dwindling reserves of essential minerals, vitamins and enzymes that were not present in your food. Again, like any stress if this were the exception your body could rebound and recover. However for many of us this is the norm, every day, for a lifetime.

So the cycle continues for days, months and years. Nutritionally empty, calorie inflated, mineral and vitamin deficient foods create liver and pancreas exhaustion, fat accumulation and rising inflammation. The burden of resistance continues to accumulate, deficiencies progress to eventual organ and system exhaustion. How long do you think the body can continue on this path? For some it will manifest as a slow malaise of fatigue and pain. For others, based upon genetics and personal constitution, it will take longer and will present itself once a disease process is fully created. Rest assured that matter what your special strengths in time the systems will always fail. So what happens when the systems begin to fail? We of course give these failures names to identify what systems are most impacted. If the sugar management component breaks down first we call this diabetes or pre-diabetes. If the body's inability to handle fat is the first to go, or the accumulation is great we call it atherosclerosis, or we monitor triglycerides, cholesterol and inflammation levels and call it cardiovascular disease. If the inflammation level gets out of control we can see chronic pain, fibromyalgia, thyroid disorders, as well as cardiovascular disease. Or perhaps your weakness is the immune system and the long-term inflammation has disabled you body's ability to identify YOUR cells from foreign cells so now an autoimmune disease manifests, like lupus, rheumatoid arthritis or polymyalgia rheumatic.

Or perhaps the deficiency and toxicity has accumulated to the level that it has affected your DNA of the cells in your body and the immune system. Now instead of cancer cells being identified by your immune system (cancer = your body's cells changing, growing out of control and no longer being a part of the community of cells in your body) and destroyed, they are not contained and spread to various areas of your body and eventually overtake all systems and cause death. This is called metastasis.

Or maybe in your case the toxins and deficiencies manifest in the central nervous system and affect the ability of the nervous to communicate, replicate and heal, so we see diseases like Parkinson's, Alzheimer's, MS and ALS.

For some, sadly, these toxins came directly into their blood stream from a multiple dose toxic exposure from a vaccination, pesticide or herbicide exposure through the skin. Perhaps they were only hours old? If they were one of the ones who could not process the load of poisons that came all at once, the resulting damage may have stunted brain development to various degrees. Some of these symptom profiles we give a new name called autism or some variant thereof. Is it possible we are creating some of these neuro-destructive disorders from our toxic exposures?

Perhaps you are one of the lucky ones and have a strong genetic composition and can process these affecters better then others, or your exposure has been very gradual, so instead of whole system effects, you experience low grade deficiencies and imbalances from your body's inability to find equilibrium. Instead of cancer, or chronic inflammation, which can cause heart disease and other more significant illness, you may have subtle dysfunction manifestations like restless leg syndrome, muscle cramping, arrhythmias or digestive dysfunction, annoying and mysterious signs that your body cannot maintain its state of health and balance.

For many reading this book this may be the first time you have considered that the common diseases in our society are partially or fully self-created. As shocking as it may seem, we all have a part in the conditions we experience. This statement will make many people angry! Do any of us choose to create disease? Most of us do not. However, if a person is a smoker and gets lung cancer, as sad as it is, there is a cause and effect which that person is responsible for. What angers most people is they do not understand that many of the things we expose ourselves to, from excess, deficiencies or toxicity, are creating an environment that greatly increases our likelihood of experiencing a disease.

It is important to understand that the body can and will heal itself when the environment supports its ability to do so. If it cannot regain balance the damage becomes permanent. The good news is, no matter what the condition, when a new environment within your body is created by you, all disease processes can be affected positively by some degree. With this new understanding many people will become overwhelmed and do one of two things. They will either say, "Screw it, I am doomed anyway" and change nothing, or will become overzealous, change everything for a short while and then quit because the change cannot be sustained.

The greatest success always occurs through consistency, so to gain control of toxicity, surplus or deficiency it is encouraged that your start slow and build upon a foundation of understanding which progresses to small actions. These small actions will lead to larger actions, consistent new actions will create in time new results, ones different then you are now experiencing. If these regular actions take away stress, healing begins to occur. It is important to remember that health and disease are both created in the same way, i.e., small daily and regular choices leading to health, or small daily and regular choices leading to disease.

Remember back to when you where taught to read, the teacher started you with the absolute basics of reading. Similarly, if we chose to live a healthier live free of disease, we must start with the basics. Start by paying attention and building from there.

Paying attention to food is done in the same way as paying attention to the thoughts in your head. Write it down, write down what goes into your mouth on a daily basis, start paying attention to what may or may not be contributing to your health and/or disease experience.

The same notebook you are using to pay attention to your thought patterns can also be used on a daily basis to write down what you eat, drink and swallow (usually medications) on a daily basis. Again, we spoke earlier about simplifying everything into one of two categories: 1. This creates health or healing or 2. It creates resistance and stress. This same process can be applied to the food we consume. As you write down what you eat on a daily basis you can determine whether what you are eating (based upon your new understanding of food and its capacity to restore or deplete) is adding to your level of health or taking away from it. As simple as it is, this exercise creates without effort a trend towards making more choices that will begin to restore balance to the systems of your body. Below is a general outline of the trends that remove or reduce nutritional stress from your body and will begin to promote health.

**Reduce:**
- Alcohol
- Sugar and flour based products
- Processed (packaged) food, fast foods
- High sugar fruits, especially bananas, grapes, oranges
- Caffeine, coffee or black tea (limit - one cup day), herbal tea not included
- Limit dairy - one serving per day
- Avoid juice, soda (especially diet drinks)

**Increase:**
- Drink water, minimum of half your body weight in ounces, i.e., 120 lbs, drink 60 ounces of water
- Eat four to six times per day. The body needs to be fed throughout the course of the day. Never skip breakfast.
- Eat at least three serving of protein per day (fish, chicken, beef, tofu, beans, eggs, etc.). Serving size is approximately the size of the center of your palm, four

to eight ounces. Protein helps keep blood sugar level since it does not create the insulin affect (see below).

-Eat a minimum of five servings of vegetables per day, and if you are hungry throughout the day eat vegetables.

-Reduce fruit intake, two or less servings per day. Although full of vitamins and antioxidants, they are high in sugar, thus most people do not eat vegetables, but instead mostly fruit. Remember veggies have more good stuff than fruit without all the simple sugar. Remember…sugar makes fat. Blood sugar rises, insulin raises, sugar is transformed into triglycerides (fat), fat stored, blood sugar drops, cravings for sugar occur and the dangerous cycle continues. This creates a condition called metabolic syndrome, which creates heart disease and diabetes.

-Fruits with lower sugar content (glycemic index), berries, watermelon, apples, etc. are preferred, however two serving per day maximum when you eat a minimum of four servings of vegetables.

-Maximum one serving of dairy per day (milk, cheese, etc). Dairy contains more fat than we need and has a high likelihood of causing an allergic response. This means it creates histamine, an allergic response that does not necessarily mean you are lactose intolerant, rather, it means histamine creates inflammation, congestion of sinus cavities and a body stressor.

- Consume one to two servings of nuts or seeds per day; serving = ¼ cup. This is great for a snack; however, it is very easy to eat one to two cups without even noticing. Nuts seeds have healthy fat and protein.

Get a reference journal. Write down everything that goes in your mouth, every day. A recent study by the Journal of Nutrition showed that people who write down what they consume get results.

Paying attention brings about change. Food is one thing most of us never pay attention to until a problem or disease arises. This is usually after decades of not paying attention, so common sense would tell us if I want to gain control of what has previously been out of control I must start paying attention. Being aware is one way to be observant, however for a person who has never considered food as one of the causes of disease, awareness is not enough. Writing things down helps to make our awareness concrete, this will help ingrain new habits. And of course our memory is always subject to our infamous justifier, you know what I am talking about, "Oh I didn't do too bad," or "I deserve this or that because I had a hard day." When we write it down we can look at the facts of our habits without our mind justifying why we did what we did.

Above is a general guide that will suit most people's body types and can be varied upon needs. Athletes and people who are physical most of the day would require modifications. However, the above guide when slowly implemented over four to six weeks accomplishes two of the major goals that are required to aid you in becoming healthy. 1. Reducing unnecessary calories and 2. Reducing toxic accumulation from the most common food sources that stress the liver, kidneys and digestive tract. Remember, stress is stress, no matter its source. The body's response is the same whether stress comes from your mind (thoughts), food/medication/chemical exposure (breathing, skin exposure etc.) or physical, the spine, the nerves, the bones or the muscles (more to come on this).

**HOW TO START**

At our clinic we use the HALF RULE, as a way to begin trending towards a new habit. The half rule is simple. You didn't create your habits, which can potentially create your death overnight, and therefore you cannot undo them overnight. If you expect a total change in direction from one day to the next failure is assured. Sadly, most can never make true change because this understanding has not been grasped. Lasting change in your life's habits take time. This statement will save you a lot of pain and frustration when you remember that persistence is the key.

THE HALF RULE: From the list of foods to avoid, cut whatever you are eating from the avoid list in half for one to two weeks, continue cutting in half the foods on the avoid list by half each week after that. Remember there is no big hurry unless you are suffering from the end stage of a chronic disease like heart disease or cancer. If this is the case you have lost the luxury of time and the change above will have to be immediate and dramatic in an effort to allow a quick health change.

For the rest of us, plan that over six to 12 months you will change your life, your health and of course by default, your physical body. Keep working on the half rule and then begin adding one of the items on the INCREASE list each week (or every second week if you decide). So you have reduced some form of stressor from the AVOID list and you have added one thing from the INCREASE list. Continue to do this the majority of the time.

**Summary:**

Nutrients are required to heal. Many foods do not contain what we need, especially in today's modern fast paced, genetically modified and highly processed world. Most of us have huge amounts of excess energy (fat storage), with absolute deficiency of what the body needs to become healthy (protein, healthy fat, nutrients that build and heal). The biggest mystery to most people is the response to stress. The food and chemicals we are exposed to, as well as the thoughts that consume our minds and our physical body functions, create responses within every cell. The strain or the support each action creates will affect our body's ability to heal and repair. Food is only one of the factors we must address as we look into health. Remember calorie restriction cannot work as a means of health restoration, and disease will always result when we are ignorant to the laws of nutritional quality and its creation of stress.

Understanding the mechanisms of how food and life create stress is the key to building understanding, which can lead to successive changes in daily patterns. How, what and when we eat gives us the means to stop the daily damage created from deficiency, toxicity and calorie overload.

Recall again, stress responses from any source (physical, mental, chemical/nutritional) create hormone changes. Hormone changes from stress (adrenal hormones) will dictate what your body can do to make energy, how it regulates blood sugar and whether it's even possible to get energy from fat storage or muscle. Therefore, diet and reducing toxic exposure from any source is one part of the answer to regaining control of the factors that create disease and suffering.

# 5

---

# The "Physical World" and Our Body

---

IT'S VERY DIFFICULT TO DRIVE YOUR CAR WITH YOUR EMERGENCY BRAKE ON!!

Think about how much energy it takes to drive a car when the emergency break was accidentally left on. Your motor is working so hard, the engine is revving, the fuel consumption is at its absolute max, every system of that car is at full capacity, yet where are you going? Nowhere, of course! The physical resistance on that vehicle is so great very little forward motion can occur. That is physical resistance at its best.

Many people do not make the connection of the basic laws of physics and our body. However, we are subject to the same physical effects as every other part of nature. Think about gravity, friction and mechanical efficiency. These are all forces our body has to contend with every single moment of every single day for a lifetime. Could you imagine that these forces over time can affect our body and eventually create resistance? Do you think in time enough strain and resistance can build and eventually compromise our overall health? You guessed it, it can and it does!

Imagine a kid carrying a huge backpack. Take a look the next time you drive by a local school. What impact do you think this backpack may have on his or her system? First of course you have the muscle impact, the fatigue, and then we have the spinal effects on the discs, ligaments and finally, the nervous system, the central controller of every cell tissue and organ in the body. How do you imagine these daily physical stressors will impact this child's spine, their growth, their development, their ability to work, sleep, and function? Now imagine this child plays sports, and perhaps they have had a few injuries, or had a car accident sometime in their life. Do you believe that the accumulation of these incidences could impact the overall function of this child's body? Gravity, strain, friction, the physical forces of nature are all influencing us, all of the time. We may not see their effects today, but we always see them later. We discussed earlier the effects of food, and how long-term unhealthy food intake can create diseases like heart disease, or cancer or diabetes. What do we call the long-term negative effects from the physical strains of life? We call it arthritis, chronic muscle pain, headaches, disc disease and nerve irritation.

Most are unaware of the cumulative effects of physical life until they feel it. Mrs. Jones, I am sorry to inform you that your hip is worn out; we will need to do a hip replacement. Sir, you have sciatica, you will need to be on this anti-inflammatory until the pain goes away, and by the way it's more than likely going to return. But, doctor, what caused it? Oh, it's just age, is the typical answer. Wrong, age is not the cause of these conditions. The cause is accumulation of life's injuries and their impact on your bones, muscles and nerves. This is great news! The ailments you "think" you have to experience as you age can be avoided if you take a few simple steps "now" to counteract the physical forces on your body. Remember STRESS? When balance cannot be maintained, damage or diseases must occur. When the efficiency of your physical machine becomes inefficient, imbalance and disease must result, its cause and effect, like putting your cold finger on a hot stove, the heat must transfer from the hot to the cold.

Does this mean we should do nothing at all? Of course not, since remaining the same ensures a continuation of the same result. The point is: Everything in life is cumulative, the effects of our daily thinking, the effects of our daily consuming or exposing and the effects of our daily physical doings. This newfound knowledge allows us to engage in new regular "UNDOINGS" to counter what we create by living. This has been written by all of the mystics and is represented as the balance many of us are familiar with, YIN AND YANG, construction and destruction, the action with no action, the doing with being. Every part of our life is a representation of the two opposing forces of nature. However, most of us are unaware and therefore we do not implement the balancing force or repair, we simply through unawareness keep breaking down. This creates results, some we like, but for most a lot of what we do not like.

So what is the answer to the ageless question: "How Do We Counter Physical Stress?"

The answer is a bit anticlimactic because you already know what it is. It's the same as the solution to gaining control of mental and nutritional stress. First, you pay attention. Observe your habits. Are you hunching and slouching, are you always in the car, or at the desk, how do the muscles feel in the back of your neck and low back? When you look in the mirror are your shoulders even or is one side higher or lower than the other? When you put your hands on your waist and look at yourself or someone else are they level or are they crooked? When you look at yourself or others from the side, where is your head, is it on top of your spine and shoulders or is it in front? If it is in front what's holding it on, is it sitting on top of the spine or hanging on the muscles of the neck? How do your shoulders feel when you touch them? Is one of them sore and achy and the other not, or are both sore? How about your hips and knees? When you exercise is one side of your body more flexible than the other? Why would one side of your body be working differently than the other? Aren't they supposed to be working the same? What happens when the one that is working harder finally gives up? Is this normal or just common?

These are the questions you need to ask yourself in order to "pay attention." If you look you "will" see there are reasons that your body is working out of balance. These imbalances over time "create" the physical conditions our elderly tell us. "If ONLY I knew, I would have done something differently." Our elderly have much to teach us with this statement, if only we would listen.

So what can we do differently? First, we pay attention. Second, we will need some help from a professional who is an expert in the world of biomechanics. These specialists, called chiropractors, can help determine what is going on with our physical system, your nerves, your muscles, your bones and joints, and how they impact the organs and systems of the body. A chiropractor will be essential for helping you find the best path to undo what life's daily physical events have created.

Remember we all create our own problems, not on purpose of course, but through the daily accumulation of life. You will want to take advantage of a biomechanical, muscular and neural specialist - your chiropractor - to help you to become proactive, instead of reactive to the forces of gravity, friction and degeneration.

So how does physical stress create resistance that our bodies then must attempt to counter? Imagine again, we all have a bucket of energy. Each person may have more or less energy in their bucket than others. The bucket represents what is available to us. On that bucket is a line, for our purposes let's call this line a threshold. It can be anywhere on that bucket, for some it's higher or lower than for others. We can call this line symptoms for some or disease for others, or any other effect of the body's inability to maintain balance.

Now, imagine all of the stressors in our life put holes in that bucket and the energy used by our body to maintain balance drops. On the contrary we also do things that plug some of those holes or add "energy" to the bucket. For instance, you are learning something new and implement new activities like reading this book, or you have a healthy habit that supports or reduces the strain on your systems. This adds more energy. If you stay above this individual threshold as we spoke of earlier, you will experience more of the effects of balance, meaning your body will be generally functional, you would have few symptoms and your likelihood of disease is lower than it would be if you were at or below the threshold line. The further or closer you are from that line in either direction would increase or decrease your experience of health. If you were near the top of the bucket your body systems are at ease, you would function efficiently. When temporary challenges show up physically, mentally or chemically/nutritionally, your body would contend with them easily and quickly, and would then return to a balanced state. Your good health would then continue. On the contrary, if you were below that balance threshold, any new stressor to the system would drive you further into imbalance.

So people ask, what causes disease? The simple answer is, imbalance to the point at which your body cannot maintain its ability to function. When break down exceeds build up, destruction always occurs. Sounds too simple they say, "My doctor told me I have a very rare and complicated form of disease," or that "My heart condition is due to high cholesterol and genetics," the complexities go on and on. Your doctors are right. The intricacies of disease are complicated, the causes are simple. Remembering from the analogy above, each person's bucket has a few factors you cannot control; we call them constitutional factors. These factors are individually dependent, genetics, epigenetics, general resilience, etc. We see these constitutional factors in all groups of people. A common example of this is the Native Americans' lower tolerance to metabolize alcohol, a Caucasian female's propensity for gallbladder dysfunction, and an African American's higher than average incidence of heart disease. These are constitutional factors affecting genetically linked groups of people, between families, and factors specific to each individual's ability to adaptable or resist the many stressors that come with life.

The factors we cannot control bring us further from the imbalance line if they are weakness, as discussed above. If these factors are constitutional strengths then we will resist or adapt and remain at a state of more balance. This is why some people can maintain balance in spite of habits or activities that speed up the destruction of the body, while others have very little resistance. We cannot deny certain individuals and groups have tendencies that can make us more or less prone to a condition, however most of us mistake this propensity to the cause, and therefore write off their power to change the course of their health and their life. This is best demonstrated in the statement, "My condition is genetic"!

How sad! As a physician I hear people every day giving up their power to change because they have been "sold" an idea that health is written in their genetics. We can see the absurdity of the statement, "I grew up without money, and therefore I will be poor." If this were true of course America would not exist, and the caste system of old Europe would remain in place. Is our health any different? We must agree that if you grew up without financial means you would have a larger distance to travel to gain large financial goals, like if you grew up with an unhealthy pattern of living. But, this does not mean it is not possible to create a different outcome from how they were raised if that is what they truly desire.

My observation is that we are all very attached to our ways of living, which is certainly understandable. That being said, the hope and purpose of this book is to help all of us evaluate our "ways" and determine if how we live is supporting where we say we want to go or is it taking us further away. So where do we want to go? In the last 22 years I have observed that everyone wants variations of the same things, to be healthy and happy. Everyone may have a different variety of health and happy, however, the attainment is the same for all of us.

### The 3$^{rd}$ Step In Becoming Happy and Healthy!

Physical stressors accumulate, they affect the muscles, they create fatigue and they create inflammation and compensation from other parts of the body. In time discs break down, the ability to manage gravity decreases, tissues (muscles, tendons, ligaments) lose their ability to adapt, spinal bone positions become altered and inefficient, nerve and nerve roots (nerves coming out of the spine) become mechanically (from the bones, muscles, ligament etc.) or chemically (from the foods, chemicals and the chemicals produced by dominant thought processes) altered. The communication between the brain and all of the systems become inefficient, responses to keep balance are slowed, the resistance rises, and the body is running full out using all of its resources like the car with the emergency brake on, huge amounts of your life energy are being exhausted and you are going nowhere. In this very common scenario healing and returning to a state of efficiency and balance cannot occur. So we continue backwards, small day-to-day issues become major complications that create disease, all arising from the simple and common unawareness of the laws of cumulative stress and the creation of imbalance.

**How to Fill Your Energy Bucket**

As we discussed earlier, this knowledge allows the opportunity for new action. A general understanding of the process of balance and a few regular consistent habits and voila, you shift from a path of disease to a path of health. Consider again, every thought, word and action either increases or decreases the level of energy in our bucket of life. The net effect is your life; it is exactly what you are experiencing in your life right now. If you like what you have, keep doing what you are doing and if you don't, you have the power to change your mind, which will change your words and of course change your actions. This is how you change your life.

Knowing how gravity creates physical stress and beginning a simple regular exercise regimen like yoga, tai chi, walking, hiking, biking, etc. helps build strength, flexibility and adaptability to the physical stressors of life. This is one way to add life energy to your "bucket."

Change your workstation, so it's more ergonomic, put the seat back up in your car and raise the rear view mirror, sleep on your side or back with a pillow between the knees. Look at yourself in the mirror and evaluate your shoulders and your hips. Ask yourself if they look the same or are off-balance. Feel the muscles of your neck and low back. Feel your hips, knees and feet, your forearms and shoulders; are they different are they the same? Look at yourself from the side, or have someone else look at you. Is your head in front of your shoulders, does your low back have a large or perhaps no curve at all? Ask yourself what this means. See a chiropractor, like you would a dentist "regularly." They can help stop and/or undo the effects of injury to the muscles, spinal bones, discs and nervous system. This will improve or restore function to the organ systems that will help you adapt to life's events. All of these simple inexpensive steps will bring you closer to balance and further and further away from imbalance and disease.

# 6

## The Big Picture

Sadly, people are often so perplexed by the variation of health and disease. "Doctor, why did this happen to me?" "What did I do wrong?" "Am I being punished? We hear these comments every day, which to me is a cry for understanding. You do not feel helpless if you have a basic understanding of cause and effect. We do not question a higher power or feel helpless when we place our hand on a hot stove and we get burned. Fire and hand equals burn and pain, which is pretty simple to equate because the effect is so close to the cause. Our body however, due to its complex nature to survive, opens the gap between cause and effect, and when you do this a delay between cause and effect is created. This confuses many of us; we then believe we did not have a hand in the cause.

If you look around, the formula is very simple. The bigger the gap between cause and effect, the greater the confusion! This is certainly evident as it applies to health and disease. It's evident elsewhere too. Look around, does this confusion exist elsewhere the confusion that comes from space between cause and effect? Look at our schools, our children, our education system. Does this apply to societal challenges as well as individual health conditions? I challenge you to ask yourself, do our actions as an individual, a group, a society or country create the experiences we are living.

It has been said by many enlightened people that if you want to change the world you must first start by changing your inner world, meaning you must change yourself. To me this means that we have very little power to change our outer environment until we change our inner environment. For instance, if we desire the outer experience of health and vitality we must create the internal environment of health and vitality. This of course begins with the smallest part of us, our individual cells. The individuals that make up the whole must have what they need to thrive. If they do not then the whole (you) cannot thrive. So the circle is complete. What's good for the goose is good for the gander. What is good for each individual cell will by default create what is good for the whole organism, YOU. It must start from the smallest part of you and in time it will progress to the entire you (your body). Is this not how disease is created, accumulation of mental/emotional, nutritional/chemical, physical/structural resistance to the point where the individual part of you, your cell could no longer maintain its equilibrium? The balance shifted, perhaps slowly over many years or quickly due to a barrage of resistance or stress coming from many sources. However it came, the downward trend allowed the experience of disease.

*Long term resistance to life = disease, unhappiness, suffering and pain.*

If resistance creates our unhappiness and the experience of what we do not desire, then of course going with the flow of life must create health, happiness and growth. In my observation this is demonstrated best if you are a gardener. How often have you lamented over the seeds you have sown? You may anxiously await the sprout to push through the soil or be hyper vigilant and over water. You know the scenario: the seed has no awareness of your internal feelings whether it is anxiousness or peace. The seed follows its own energetic connection to the cycle of life. You give it the environment it needs and it will thrive. Water, soil and sunlight are for the most part all it needs to follow its cycle and produce the fruit it was destined to produce. Introduce along the way resistance to its process and you will alter its ability to manifest its perfect nature. Your worry, fret and frustration will create inappropriate, unnecessary and possibly negative actions that will actually prevent or slow down the seeds' inborn capacity to thrive. From my observation we are much the same as the plant, thus the answer to some of our deepest frustrations regarding our health and perhaps our deepest life frustrations can be undone, avoided and healed. How can this occur? By restoring our faith back into our body. Like our faith in the seed, within it is the coding to not only survive but THRIVE, if we simply avoid a few simple barriers that will hinder its natural ability to grow.

Once we know what these resistors are we can simply trend away from them like we would avoid too much sun or overwatering of our garden. Check out the list below. There you will find a couple of the mental stressors that can prevent you from getting where you want to go. The hope is for us to look at the list, like a new gardener would read a book on how to raise a healthy garden. With this intention we can begin to implement the elements that create the outcome we desire and steer away from those that do not.

Mental resistors to life's natural state of health:
-Unexpressed and repressed anger
-Resentment
-Belief systems that are limiting to life (I am better than, you are less than, I am not good enough or smart enough, the world is bad, people are bad, etc.)
-Judgment of self, which results in judgment of others
-Lack of faith, need to control

# 7

## An Easy Reader's Guide to Changing Your Life

**Summary: Gaining control of stress from the mind**

-Think about what you are thinking about.

-Journal, in time your beliefs will emerge, opening the opportunity for you to decide if this belief or that is valid, if it holds true to filling you with peace keep it, if it does not you may consider cultivating a new perspective, which in time will change your belief.

-Add new input like you are doing with this book. Read, go to a yoga class, pray, meditate, go to church if that attracts you, get to know people who you admire or who have mastered what you desire. New input into your mind allows perspectives on life to be altered, much like reading allows the reader to learn about things they may never actually experience. Embracing a new understanding through the words or the company of those who have created what you desire will change your vantage point. And open your mind and change your beliefs of what is possible for you, as this will change your actions.

-Observe your feelings, happy, sad, angry, joyful, indifferent, uptight and anxious. Feelings direct you to your beliefs; journaling helps you pay attention to your overall level of allowing. For example we all have our topics which create heated resistance:  For some it's same-sex marriage, for others divorce or political viewpoints. The list is endless; however the reason for the resistance is always the same, a strong judgment regarding this topic. The stronger the anger and the more numerous the topics of your anger the more stress you are creating. The greater the internal stress the larger the effect on the body and its systems. Does that mean we should all endorse and support behaviors and lifestyles that we do not agree with? The obvious answer of course is no, however accepting is not endorsing, it is choosing to not allow something to affect you, even if you have a deep desire to change it.

Marianne Williamson has written that no amount of feeling bad can help someone else. If my feeling bad about something could help you or me, then by all means we should feel bad. However, that is not possible and the only way to help myself and therefore help someone else is to change perspective.

This of course is the premise behind the art of forgiveness. Forgiveness does not mean you give others permission to continue to damage you. Forgiveness has little to do with those who have in some way injured you. Rather, it is purely an act to support YOUR survival and restore YOUR PEACE and remove resistance to your natural flow of growth and health. Forgiveness is the process of embracing the idea that I CHOOSE to no longer allow YOUR actions to hurt me by my continual remembrance and cyclical reiteration of the past. Forgiveness is a purely SELFISH act, which is essential to restore peace to YOU. Most reading that statement would say to be selfish is bad, because we have heard that to focus on yourself is arrogant, however if you consider forgiveness it is a truly enlightened SELFISH act of restoring SELF to peace, and removing others' power over you through past acts. Therefore, we can understand how forgiveness can become one of the antidotes to the stress we create in our minds, one of the dominant causes of disease in our body. When we implement the art of selfishness, meaning the art of putting your attention on yourself, rather than putting your attention on others, you can gain a handle on the causes of resistance, the resistance that when left uncontrolled will add up to disease.

Again, this is counter to what we are taught. We have been taught we must put our attention on others, but what control do we have over anyone other than ourselves? We can support, encourage and help others, yet we have no real control over anyone other than ourselves. Therefore if we begin paying attention to ourselves, looking after ourselves, creating more peace within our minds, not only will our internal environment change, our immune system will strengthen, our cell environment will begin to heal, our body will strengthen and of course our outer environment will change. Can you imagine how your relationships will improve when you love yourself, and how much abundance you have to give to others? If you want to change the world you must change yourself. It appears that this would be a difficult endeavor. However, if you consider the effects of not changing, the choice becomes clear. There is always a small amount of discomfort from embracing new ideas, but it is always less in the long run.

Remember from earlier chapters, we do not create conditions on purpose; conditions are outcomes of imbalance. When our body and for that matter our mind cannot maintain balance between the building up and the breaking down from life's stressors, systems fail. How many and how much depends on the degree of imbalance, when systems fail, a myriad of conditions which doctors around the world name and spend a great deal of time attempting to cure. This of course is a fine, necessary and noble task, essential for us all to understand if we desire to have control over what the Health vs. Disease experience is. We must first become conscious of this buildup break down process, and then take small regular actions as a result of this new awareness.

Awareness without change is simply trivia and has little value. I have observed in many years of practice that people know a lot. They have a great deal of knowledge as a result of the Internet, television and access to everything. This is great; however few ever make real changes in spite of having the tools at their fingertips. Knowledge is not enough. Awareness is not enough. Awareness which leads to action builds the foundation to change your life. This is where the links for change are usually broken, people do not know how to or where to start. The gap between where you find yourself now and where you want to be is so great you do not know where to begin. You try by sheer will, you push and after several days or for some several weeks you give up, get distracted and go back to what you know. These are the behaviors you have always had, the ones you have had since you were a child, the behaviors you embraced as a mechanism to cope with the trials and tribulations of your life, the ones you learned and have gotten you this far. What is different now? Your awareness and your expectation; which when combined with small regular changes and persistence, the chain of change can be constructed.

## Summary: Reducing your Stress load

Food, air, water, pharmaceuticals, skin and hair care products, household cleaners, plastics, paint and lawn care are all suspects that accumulate in our body. If it has chemicals in it, these chemicals add stress to our system. We all need to be aware and REDUCE our exposure when we can. The purpose of this book is to help us to become aware of, and to reduce and gain control of what we can, giving our body more ability to adapt to what we can't. The simple take home is, change your food for the better, improve the air quality of your home and become conscientious of what you can control, to give your body the chance to heal and diseases to stop.

**Food:**
 **Reduce:**
- Alcohol
-Sugar and flour based products
-Processed (packaged) food, fast foods
-High sugar fruits, especially bananas, grapes, oranges
-Caffeine, coffee or black tea (limit-1 cup day), herbal tea not included
-Limit dairy - one serving per day
-Avoid juice, soda (especially diet drinks)

**Increase:**
-Drink water, minimum of half your body weight in ounces, i.e., 120 lbs, drink 60 ounces of water.

-Eat four to six times per day. The body needs to be fed throughout the course of the day. Never skip breakfast.

-Eat at least three serving of protein per day, (fish, chicken, beef, tofu, beans, eggs, etc.). Serving size is approximately the size of the center of your palm, four to eight ounces. Protein helps keep blood sugar level since it does not create the insulin effect (see below).

-Eat a minimum of five servings of vegetables per day, and if you are hungry throughout the day eat vegetables.

-Reduce fruit intake to two or less servings per day. Although full of vitamins and antioxidants, they are high in sugar, thus most people eat mostly fruit rather than vegetables. Remember, veggies have more good stuff than fruit without all the simple sugar. Sugar makes fat. Blood sugar rises, insulin raises, sugar is transformed into triglycerides (fat), fat stored, blood sugar drops, cravings for sugar occur and the dangerous cycle continues. This creates a condition called metabolic syndrome, which creates heart disease and diabetes.

-Fruits with lower sugar content (glycemic index), berries, watermelon, apples, etc. are preferred, however, consume two serving per day maximum when you eat a minimum of four servings of vegetables.

-Maximum one serving of dairy per day (milk, cheese etc). Dairy contains more fat than we need and has a high likelihood of causing an allergic response. Which means it creates histamine, an allergic response does not necessarily mean you are lactose intolerant, it means histamine creates inflammation, congestion of sinus cavities and is a body stressor.

-One to two servings of nuts or seeds per day, serving ¼ cup. Nuts and seeds are great for a snack, however it is very easy to eat one to two cups without even noticing. Nuts and seeds have healthy fat and protein.

NEVER EVER use artificial sweeteners, Splenda/aspartame, etc. These are neurotoxic compounds (poisonous to your nerves), create free radicals and although they have no calories they have been shown to suppress your body's ability to metabolize fat.

## Non-Organic Foods vs. Organic Foods

Pesticides, herbicides, food waxes, hormones, antibiotics and genetically modified plant proteins are readily found in our non-organic food supply. There is a great deal of talk these days about organic versus non-organic food sources. A lot of people think it is just hype; however I urge them to look into this debate further. If we only ate once week or once a month, the urgency becomes less paramount, however most of us eat several times per day for our entire lifetime. Their effects accumulate quickly. That is why we look at food and water as the two most important daily events that can add to or take away from the creation of disease.

I will encourage everyone reading these pages to first make an effort to consume only organic meats, fishes, eggs and dairy (although dairy should be avoided). Once you have made that switch then work on eliminating non-organic fruits and vegetables. Why change animal based foods first? Simply, because animals are most like humans and what affects their growth and function will definitely affect our growth and function. We always want to change what will cause the most damage first.

## Water

Make water your primary beverage. Aim for half of your body weight per day in ounces. If you weigh 150lbs your goal is 75 ounces per day (1/2 of 150). If you are physical during the day or it is hot drink more. Most people do not drink water when it isn't around them or they have to go somewhere to get it. Make water available, have a refillable bottle by your desk, in your car, in the kitchen, and remember if it's around, you will more likely drink it. If you wait until you are thirsty it's too late, you are already dehydrated, which means your metabolic stress level is higher than it needs to be.

## Plastics

Avoid using plastics when you can, they leach into your food, which of course gets into your body. Consider food storage in glass containers like Pyrex. Avoid disposable water bottles and consider reusable glass or BPA free plastic, NEVER microwave in plastic and make a best effort to avoid freezing foods in plastic.

It has become common knowledge that the chemicals in plastic act like hormones in men, women and children and can create diseases associated with hormone conditions, not to mention certain types of cancer.

## Household Cleaners

Want a natural clean without the toxic load to your lungs, liver and skin? Try rubbing alcohol for the hard surfaces. Rubbing alcohol removes grease and fat like a charm. 50/50 vinegar and water works well on counters, wood, showers and other surfaces. Remember harsh chemical cleaners work well, however when you spray it you breathe it in. When you get it on your skin it breaks down the natural fatty protective layers of your skin and gets right into your blood stream. These chemicals add up, and are a challenge to the liver, not to mention that these chemicals have been known to cause certain types of headaches.

## Hair Care, Skin Care

If you spray it on know it will end up in your lungs, if you apply it to your body, it we definitely end up in your blood stream. This is an important fact, if it's safe to eat then putting in your hair or on your skin is a reasonable idea. Look into natural products. Though they may not hold your hair in place as well or smell as fragrant, consider the lifetime impact. If I can reduce the chemical toxicity of my body in an effort to reduce my risk of chronic disease, is it worth it to me? When I ask patients this question once they are experiencing a disease they will always say YES. However the power to gain as much change as they want is often lost. The power of change is best accomplished prior to the disease. Sound dramatic? Talk to someone who is experiencing a chronic disease that could have been prevented! I don't know one lung cancer patient who doesn't wish they stopped smoking sooner.

## Pharmaceuticals

Little needs to be said here, we all know medications serve a purpose and are chemically based. These foreign chemicals create toxic stress to our body, though they serve a purpose, in most cases they are not a long-term solution. It will be important to stay aware of the fact that very few medications prevent disease and even fewer cure. Their primary role is to manage symptoms, which always comes at a cost of creating more strain on one's already deteriorating systems. Use them wisely with a plan in reduce and eventually get off the medications. In most cases this is possible; the first step will be following the steps in this book and making new consistent habits. Second, talk to your prescribing doctor once you have implemented the changes in this book for a minimum of three months and physical changes begin to occur. The key to your success is consistency. That being said, if you change your body by making it healthy, and have the habits to prove and the lab tests to verify your success, your prescribing doctor may eliminate the medications you are taking.

## Lawn care (Choose Dandelions Over Disease)

You heard it correctly, lawn care! Remember, exposure from life-depleting chemicals comes from many sources. The purpose here is to gain control of the ones we can actually change. That perfect manicured lawn comes at a cost, to the people sitting on it or walking alongside it, and to all of us that require water to survive. Herbicide and fertilizer residue invariably impacts the chemical load of our body. Do you want dandelions and quack grass or do we want to expedite the destruction of our detoxifying organs, our liver, kidneys, colon and bladder? I encourage people to choose the dandelions over expediting disease.

**Gravity, Friction and Physical Effects of Life**
As we have all observed, life accumulates. We are all products of our habits, the ones we have created on purpose like exercise, sitting up straight, doing yoga, keeping flexible, seeing a chiropractor and the like, and the ones we have unconsciously adopted, i.e., injuries from sports, life, car accidents, posture, sleeping, etc. Earlier we summarized, "We are what we eat." That phrase can be expanded to "We are what we do." Eating is of course one of those "doings" as is moving. Moving about the world as we live, work and play, and the general function of our body also has an effect on the specific parts that are allowing us to move at all. Like the individual cells in our body, our individual parts that allow movement and support to the muscles, spine and nerves are sensitive to physical imbalance. Once again if we forget the laws of friction, gravity and compensation, physical accumulation overcomes the body's ability to sway in the wind of life. With this come the physical ailments of strain, degeneration and orthopedic based conditions of the joint, muscles, bones, nerves and connective tissues.

Few will disagree that physical symptoms are difficult to ignore. Back pain, headaches, joint pain, arthritis, Carpal Tunnel syndrome, muscular pain and disc problems are just a few of the chronic ailments which consume much of our mental energy.

Where most people fall short in overcoming their ailments is simple when you recognize that pain is hard to ignore. Thus most become distracted from the symptoms and overlook the real cause of their physical conditions. You can never get to the cause by focusing on the symptoms. We see this so clearly in our modern age of medicine. This is great if you are selling symptom relievers, but not so great if you are one of the millions searching for the causes of these debilitating conditions. So what is the first step? Let's begin.

1.  Pain is the perfect motivator; don't think for a moment that your body is somehow failing you. Pain is there to get your attention and to tell you something has gone way off course. In the short term you will need to address the symptom, since it is rather difficult to be introspective when you have a knife in your back (figuratively). Find a means to furnish some form of comfort without sacrificing other systems of your body in the process. I am always tentative to recommend anything that takes all the pain away, because human nature is such that if the symptom dissolves entirely due to a symptom reliever we fall into the "I must be better"

trap. Utilize natural pain relievers, ice, bromelain, papain, turmeric, white willow bark extract, to name a few. If pharmaceutical products are necessary use wisely, setting a plan for their quick elimination. Your medical physician can help with this process.

2. Do not fall into the infamous vortex of self-deception; my symptom is gone, I must be better, though I have changed nothing. It may be a fine idea if you are talking about a virus or bacteria or a cut on your finger, but when it comes to ongoing processes this way of thinking will lead you further off course. This will result in a further progression of a negative health experience, maybe not today but definitely in the future.

3. Start from where you are right now, not where you hope or wish you could be. If you can't walk, move your arms. If your back hurts, tighten your stomach, if you can only move your shoulder a few degrees move it a few degrees. If you can't stand straight, sit as straight as you can. If it hurts to look up, look up as much as you can. If you only have unhealthy foods available read the labels and chose the best of the lot. If you are overwhelmed with negative, pessimistic or victim-based thoughts, chose one that makes you feel lighter. You get the picture. Nature's laws and I would suppose spiritual laws prevail, "To those who have, more is given, to those

who have not, more is given also." (Author interpretation of Mathew 13:12, Mark 4:25) If you keep moving in one direction, the momentum you will create will perpetuate you in that same direction. It has to! If you do not move, more non-movement will be given, so do what you can and do it regularly, exactly where you are right now. If you are in an office, start there, if you are in a hospital bed, or anywhere in between start now and where you are.

4. Be consistent and be patient. Remember, you are a product of your habits. Habits by definition are repeated ingrained actions; mental or physical makes no difference. Whatever components of this book you wish to implement first just do it. Think about it, imagine it happening and pay attention to yourself, with the idea of continually "one-upping" yourself from the day before. Do not look too far up the road to where you want to go, or too far back to where you have been. Pick your action, such as changing what you put in your body, how you move or the thoughts you ruminate over in your mind. Take an action. Do what you can right now and do better than you did yesterday. In time the results will be recognized. Do not give up.

This is where patience comes in. Changing direction takes time and energy. Total reversing any direction which has momentum is incredibly difficult. Most people do not understand this law and therefore they fail. So you begin changing a little bit each day, a little bit more each week, even more each month, and great changes occur over the years. That is why patience is essential to your process.

5. Start one thing at a time and follow your course. A ship without a rudder has no direction. Recognize when you make a choice, you have now given yourself a rudder. You have taken a stand and have set a course; a very powerful stand if it is for positive action and very destructive if it is a non-supportive action. A healthy positive stand should be guarded from others unless they are 100 percent supportive (a doctor with these understandings can help guide you in the right direction). Through choice you have taken a stand, which is good, however most of us are riddled with insecurity, and with insecurity comes doubt. Though you make a choice you have yet to experience the benefits of a positive choice, a dangerous place for you if you allow the influence of others to sway you from your choice. I like the analogy of a new seedling planted in the garden of your mind. Being similar to a new positive action one is planting in the habits of their life (this can apply to any type of action be it, physical, mental or biochemical/food related makes no difference). A new seedling has all of the elements of a full grown healthy adult plant; however it cannot withstand the full challenge of

the elements, so you must protect it from the full sun, the pouring rain and the movement of the other creatures which are in its environment.

Our new thoughts and positive actions need this protection also. They are not ready to take on the world around you yet. Do not throw them into it or they will die, with the opinions and criticisms of others. I presume most of you reading these words can relate. How many times has a well-meaning spouse's words flushed our young growing habits, or your trusted family physician, your best friend, your family members or some expert you see on TV? Others' opinions and influences can devastate a new positive pattern, whereas a mentor, a trained physician or a guiding book like this one can help support this environment of protection until your habits become ingrained.

It is true the perspectives of others can have value and can help us define balance. However, it is my observation that most of us are products of our habitual environment of thought, word and action. If we go to that same environment for advice it is unlikely we will find support for new ideas, and thus one must be guarded. I preface this for those with a history of mental illness, anorexia, bulimia, obsessive compulsive disorders, bipolar disease etc., or for the young who read this book. Balance will require the aid of others who by example and personal health can help you define these boundaries.

# 8

## The Stress Affect and the Art of Living

So, here we are. We have covered the never-ending sway of life, the physical elements of movement, posture, muscles, bones and joints, the chemical elements of food, toxicity, detoxification and the mental elements of the prevailing thought processes that we entertain.

What next? Acceptance! Stress will never end, nor will friction/gravity or positive/negative, up/down, cold/hot, good/bad, build up/breakdown, yin/yang. The cycle of life will never stop. All that can ever change is our perceptions, and our acceptance of these dichotomies of life and the ability to be at peace with it. When we understand it and accept the laws of this world, the decisions we make can be guided by what we desire, while we take full responsibility for where we are.

Stress is destroying our health, our lives, our relationships and our children. For most this would mean that stress is bad, which is not the case. That would be like saying cold is bad, it is not bad or good it just is.

When we understand that our health is the outcome of the cumulative actions we take, we can begin taking new actions. If we like what we are experiencing in any aspect of our life than accept it. Keep doing what you are doing and recognize that you through your thoughts, words and actions have made this so. If you are unhappy with what you are experiencing, accept it and start doing something different (one of the purposes of this book), and recognize that you through your thoughts, words and actions have created this experience also.

So the purpose of this book is simple, to help us all recognize that we are creating what we experience, all of us. My hope for you is very simple, "to give you new perspectives on how we all create." As a physician I have now spent many years helping patients understand how they have created what they do not want, as it relates to their body and their health, and help them create less of the physical conditions that cause them suffering. How do we do this? By implementing the steps laid out in this book. These simple steps when taken can help anyone who has a desire to experience more health and happiness.

We spoke about constitution, your personal ability to adapt. We spoke about genetics and how one's ability to adapt may be different from one to another. These facts are all accurate, though we are all different; we are also all the same. Therefore as you have learned, taking new action will reduce stress, increase efficiency and bring your closer to health. Will these actions reverse all that ails you? One cannot say, but this is for certain, your body will function better, your internal stress level will reduce and therefore your external stress level will decline. Isn't that what it's all about, to gain peace?

The secret of all life is now unveiled. The great spiritual gurus of all time have all been saying the same thing, but few of us recognize its application to every part of our everyday lives. It is about balance: how you move, how you spend your days at work, at home, in the car, sleeping, exercising, resting, eating, fasting, eliminating, building muscles, breaking down muscles, interacting with yourself, interacting with others, thinking positive thoughts, thinking negative thoughts. All aspects of life when in balance will support growth, peace and cooperation.

This applies to both our communities, the ones within our bodies, which are made of our cells and the ones without that are made up of our neighborhoods, our cities, our countries and the world.

This never-ending balance when maintained creates the true art of living!